The Ultimate Mind/Body System for Men

9 STEPS TO BUILDING YOUR SEXUAL STAMINA

By Walter Beckley

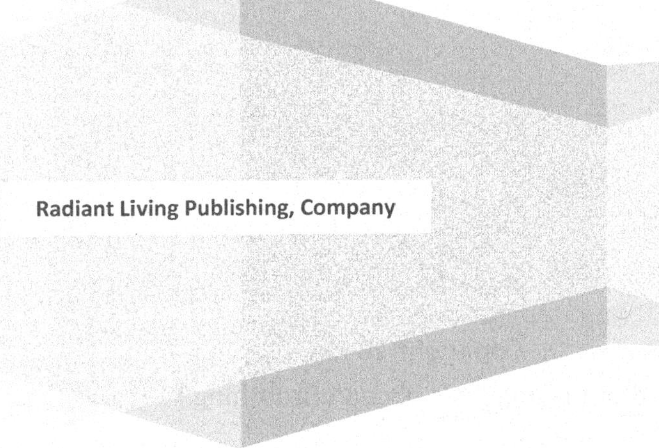

Radiant Living Publishing, Company

Congratulations. In purchasing and reading this book, you have made a wise decision. You are about to embark on a journey that will change your sexual life by giving you the most groundbreaking strategies ever discovered to improve and empower you sexually.

To gain the full benefits of this program, you need to take the following steps:

1. Read this book in its entirety.
2. Practice the exercises found in Chapters 7 to 17.
3. Join our Elite Membership site.

FOR A MORE IN-DEPTH CONNECTION AND UNDERSTANDING, HEAR AND SEE OUR AUDIO AND VIDEO SERIES

When you join our Elite Membership site, you'll gain access to our audio and video library, which will enhance your learning experience. Plus, you'll get bonus information that will enable you to become a master in the art of lovemaking.

Go to:

http://www.BuildingYourSexualStamina.com/member

START DATE ______/______/ ______/

Notes:

INDEX

Caution

This section is for my lawyers and for people who are unbalanced and seek to blame others for their shortcomings.

This book represents years of personal study with various master teachers of sex and sexual energy, as well as the practical experiences of the author.

This work is not intended to take the place of medical advice, be used as a prescription, nor is it intended to replace any drug or be viewed as a cure for any medical condition. Readers are advised to seek the advice of their personal physicians before entering into any health-related program or strategy.

The author, publisher and distributor disclaim any specific improvements, guarantees or warranties of any kind, express or implied, with regard to the pages or the information contained herein; specifically the publisher disclaims any warranties of merchantability or fitness for purpose.

PLEASE NOTE: These sexual teachings have been time tested for thousands of years in the ancient Taoist yoga, qigong (chi kung), kung fu and meditation monasteries of China as well as in the great yoga and meditation temples and Tantric schools of India.

9 Steps to Building Your Sexual Stamina is the product of more than 5,000 years of study, training and experience based on the ancient masters, seekers and kings from Ancient Kemet (Egypt), China and India.

FOR A MORE IN-DEPTH CONNECTION AND UNDERSTANDING, HEAR AND SEE OUR AUDIO AND VIDEO SERIES

When you join our Elite Membership site, you'll gain access to our audio and video library, which will enhance your learning experience. Plus, you'll get bonus information that will enable you to become a master in the art of lovemaking.

Go to:

http://www.BuildingYourSexualStamina.com/member

Take it easy and slow—and enjoy the ride—and you'll do a great work inside yourself.—Walter

ACKNOWLEDGEMENTS

I would like to acknowledge all of the seekers of greater understanding of life, health, wealth, longevity and love. May you express and experience life to its fullest in all its wildly multidimensional beauty.

I would like to thank my many students and clients who have shared so candidly with me their positive and negative experiences in life and sex. Many of their quotes and comments appear in this book, in my CDs and DVDs, on my Web sites and in my lectures.

I would especially like to thank my many teachers, who have blessed me with their knowledge and insights about the flow of energy and healing love sexology.

I would like to thank Taoist Master Mantak Chia. He has been a teacher, mentor and friend. I was certified by Taoist Master Mantak Chia to teach in 1989 under the Healing Tao System, now the Universal Tao based in Thailand.

I would also like to thank Sifu James McNeil with the Nine Little Heaven Kung Fu School for his training and advice.

Without the mentoring and example of these two principal teachers—and all that I have learned from them about the flow of energy, sexual energy, healing and movement—this book would not have been possible.

I would also like to thank Douglas Abrams Arava for his invitation to participate and contribute to his and Taoist master Mantak Chia's groundbreaking bestseller, *The Multi-Orgasmic Man*.

SPECIAL THANKS TO SO MANY BEAUTIFUL SUPPORTERS

I'd also like to thank my many helpers, helpmates and supporters for being so consistent through the years in standing by me and sharing in this work. Your assistance has been a gift and a blessing.

Many thanks go out to: John Weston, Madeline Goldstein, Patricia Davis, John Butler, Marty Doyle, Dr. Deidre Burrell, Dr. Jifunza and Fred Wright, Rosie Garcia, Dr. Morris Williamson, Larry Cherry, Luvina Beckley, Dr. Reginald Ginseng Cain and, to all of you who are not listed, please forgive me for not including your names. I do thank you from my heart to yours.

A, very special thanks to my editor James Clyde Sellman, Ph.D. for his vast knowledge and insight.

Join my teleconference classes and become involved in my Elite Membership site to learn even more and have your questions answered personal by me and my staff. —Walter

Please visit:
http://www.BuildingYourSexualStamina.com/member

FOREWORD BY GRAND MASTER MANTAK CHIA

With over 20 years of study and training, Walter Beckley is an extremely competent teacher and writer. And in this book, Walter brings out the transformational power, ease of use and essence of these once-hidden teachings.

Walter has assisted me throughout the last 20-plus years, as a Universal Healing Tao Senior Instructor and workshop coordinator. Walter is also a contributor to my bestselling book *The Multi-Orgasmic Man* and to *Chi Nei Tsang*, my book on the ancient healing arts.

It gives me great pleasure to write the forward to his new and groundbreaking book *9 Steps to Building Your Sexual Stamina: The Ultimate Mind/Body System for Men*.

9 Steps to Building Your Sexual Stamina goes straight to the heart of how to develop the sexual skills to be a great lover. Walter has developed and adapted age-old Taoist teachings on lovemaking by providing clear, step-by-step formulas and exercises, so men can easily train and channel their sexual energies—strengthening their subtle ring muscles and thus enabling them to consistently maintain their erections without taking a pill. Walter also shares a variety of concepts and methods that will enable a man to satisfy his mate over and over again.

Within *9 Steps to Building Your Sexual Stamina*, students become well-versed in the knowledge and skills required for a true mastery of lovemaking. There are five very important reasons why I believe every man should be sexually trained in this manner:

1st—Men will improve their health and vitality.

2nd—They will easily be able to maintain their erections for as long as they want.

3rd—They will be able to experience multiple orgasms.

4th—They will feel more confident and empowered.

5th—They will consistently be able to satisfy their partners.

I hope that men and women everywhere will see how important it is that men learn and become accustomed—acclimated—to these high-level skills in lovemaking. Walter's training methods will improve the quality of any relationship, simply because a well-satisfied woman makes for a harmonious household. And it will open her to deeper and more loving relationships—with herself, her mate and her family, friends and life.

In conclusion, this level of training is worth more than gold. When you understand these principles, your value as a lover will increase. Your health and vitality will improve. This science of lovemaking will make the difference that you have sought after as a man and as a lover.

—Taoist Grand Master Mantak Chia

About the Author—Walter Beckley

Walter Beckley is the founder of the School of Radiant Living. He is a dynamic speaker, trainer, healer, life coach, writer and teacher's advisor. He enjoys working with and assisting others with their physical, mental, emotional, sexual or spiritual challenges.

Walter's desire to share his love and zest for life led him down the path of helping others to discover, experience and express the power of love in their own lives. He combines the best of many different healing modalities. And his work is designed to bring vibrant balance and clarity to all aspects of life.

Walter began his official training in 1977. Due to his intense desire to expand his own life and help others uncover their own radiant, divine creative force, he studied various healing modalities in the United States and abroad.

Walter is an avid student and teacher of the energetic and spiritual connection of the mind, body and emotions. Born and raised in Joliet, Ill., his studies and teachings have led him to India, Thailand, Europe, Mexico, Brazil and the Caribbean.

Walter conducts private, group and couples' sessions; seminars; retreats; telephone consultations; and on-site business training. He also provides teacher-training certification and distributes a variety of health products.

A much-sought-after national and international speaker, Walter has appeared on numerous radio and television programs; has lectured at conferences, in auditoriums and other venues; and has contributed to numerous publications.

In addition, Walter has produced several books, music and spoken-word CDs and DVDs on how to live a more productive life, including *The Healthy Living Game Plan* book series:

- *5 Sources of Silent Toxic Killers That Attack Your Body*
- *Super Charge Your Life—Detoxify, Revitalize and Heal Your Body, Look and Feel Better in 30 Days or Less*
- *Overcoming Diabetes Naturally in 30 Days*

As well as:

- *"Focused-Power Breathing" DVD and CD*
- *"Radiant Hand-Body Activation Method" DVD, CD and VHS*
- *"Inner Body Workout" DVD*
- *"Ocean Breathing" CD*

Walter is also a contributor to two bestselling books by Mantak Chia and the Universal Tao Co.—*The Multi-Orgasmic Man* and *Chi Nei Tsang* (*Internal Healing Organ Massage*).

The goal of Walter's work is to celebrate life by teaching simple and highly effective techniques that enable others to release stress and trauma on all levels and tap into (and restore) their own radiant life force—and, in so doing, manifest their desires and create permanent, positive changes in their lives.

To: All Men Everywhere,
Master your penis, and you will heal and awaken yourself—and your lover(s).
I'll give you the best of what I've learned in all my explorations and research to insure that you excel. However, you must take the time and learn these secrets, and practice these methods in order to create the sexual stamina to become a long-lasting lover naturally, without pills, creams, herbs or other male enhancement products.
—Walter

INTRODUCTION

Congratulations! You've made one of the most important choices you'll ever make for empowering your life and improving your sexual abilities. By deciding to purchase this book and taking the time to learn its easy-to-understand, step-by-step lessons, you'll transform not just your sexual experiences but those of your partner as well. In so doing, you'll be light-years ahead of other men and their sexual abilities.

This is not a thick book, but you don't want to read an encyclopedia to learn how to improve your sexual health and performance, do you? This is a bare nuts-and-bolts kind of book. It will serve not only as a quick-start guide to your sexual capabilities, but as an invaluable aid in your quest to improve your life as a whole. As you practice the lessons of *9 Steps to Building Your Sexual Stamina*, you'll learn to expand as a person in **all** aspects of your life. And as you train your body, those lessons and experiences will take your sexual experiences—and your life—to new heights.

This is the best choice you could ever make when it comes to improving your sexual skills!
—Walter

OVERVIEW

YOU'LL LEARN 11 POWERFUL CONCEPTS DESIGNED TO INTENSIFY YOUR SEXUAL EXPERIENCE AS A MAN.

1. How to become multi-orgasmic.

2. How to experience deeper, more satisfying sex.

3. How to delay ejaculation.

4. How to have effortless self-control.

5. How to gain the freedom and confidence that will allow you to fulfill your partner's deepest desires.

6. How to attain new heights of pleasure beyond your imagination.

7. How to enhance your relationships.

8. How to improve your communication in and out of the bedroom.

9. How to become more loving, caring and considerate.

10. How to have deeper, longer-lasting sexual experiences with your partner.

11. How to deepen your partner's love for you by helping her experience and learn more about herself.

FOR A MORE IN-DEPTH CONNECTION AND UNDERSTANDING, HEAR AND SEE OUR AUDIO AND VIDEO SERIES

When you join our Elite Membership site, you'll gain access to our audio and video library, which will enhance your learning experience. Plus, you'll get bonus information that will enable you to become a master in the art of lovemaking.

Go to:

http://www.BuildingYourSexualStamina.com/member

1
SEXUAL SECRETS FOR MEN

***9 Steps to Building Your Sexual Stamina* is a unique sexual training system. Based on ancient secrets for developing sexual power, stamina, rock-hard erections and ejaculation control, this training system will help you eliminate problems with your performance as a man and enable you to become a masterful lover.** When you utilize our training methods, you and your partner will begin enjoying great sex each and every time—plus you'll get better and last longer with each encounter.

If you are less than satisfied with your sexual performance, it's important to realize that you're not alone. Men all over the world—for thousands of years—have experienced the same difficulties. And little seems to have changed: We still have major problems getting it up and keeping it up. (Just think of all those commercials for Viagra, Cialis, Levitra, etc.) Few men can control their erections, orgasms, ejaculations and overall lovemaking skills and stamina. Very few realize they can have multiple orgasms.

For more than 5,000 years, the sexual knowledge in *9 Steps to Building Your Sexual Stamina* was a well-guarded secret handed down from teacher to disciple. This training system is a modernized version of those ancient teachings about sex, sexual energy and the art of love. Following this program, you'll learn to revitalize and deepen your sexual experiences and to have better and longer-lasting sex. In short, this book offers a proactive, systematic, easy-to-use program for men who want to increase and master their sexual energy.

WHAT IS SEX?

From the biological or physical standpoint, sex or sexual intercourse, takes place when the male reproductive organ (the penis) enters into the female reproductive organ (the vagina). When a man enters a woman, they are having sex.

Having sex doesn't mean having good sex or great sex. To be able to experience great orgasmic sex that lasts for hours is a skill that a couple must master. Although this book is focused on men, remember that women, too, must learn to master their sexual muscle group.

Moreover, women's paths to orgasm vary greatly. Some women are non-orgasmic because of a difficulty that may be mental, emotional or physical. Some take a long time to reach orgasm, while others do so very quickly. Some can achieve an orgasm by crossing and rocking their legs; others, simply by thinking intensely about making love. Of course, a given woman's sexual responsiveness also varies, depending on various internal and external factors.

As you can see, women's sexual responsiveness involves a variety of factors—mind and body, internal as well as external. My next book, on female sexual vitality, will cover this subject in depth.

DON'T STRIKE OUT—GO FOR THE GOLD

When having sex, most men want to be able to please and pleasure their woman for a long time. But instead of hours, they ejaculate in a matter of minutes—without having reached the intensity they desired. Even if his partner has an orgasm, a man may feel let down at the disparity between what he'd planned to do and what actually happened. Too often, both are left unsatisfied.

For a while, a woman may accept and believe that this level of performance is enough. But her man may feel that she **deserves** more—and may sense that she **wants** more ... And what if she meets someone who truly rocks her world ... for an hour ... or more ... ? Where will he be then?

Many men have been there, with that critical voice in their heads saying, "It's a swing and a miss ... a swing and a miss ..." and worrying that they'll keep hitting pop ups and foul balls or just plain striking out—never getting that grand slam. But that's what she wants: She wants **YOU** to hit a home run. She wants **YOU** to knock it out the park.

Think of this book as your personal spring training program to get you in shape for America's **other** great pastime.

THE FOUR BASIC CATEGORIES OF MALE SEXUAL PERFORMANCE

Category #1

If you are capable of having sex for, say, 20 to 30 minutes (or more) this book will help you become a masterful and even longer-lasting lover. By the way, you should be commended for taking the time to enhance and further your sexual skills.

Category #2

If you are taking pills, using creams or taking herbal remedies to become erect or increase your stamina, this book will help you get off those male enhancement products and teach you how to enhance your lovemaking skills naturally and without risk of side effects. Armed with this book, you'll have all the ammunition you need to improve your sexual skills and become a masterful lover. And knowledge is power: As you go through our training system and gain increasing control over your lovemaking skills, you'll feel your confidence growing as well.

Category #3

If you experience erectile dysfunction as a result of health-related issues—such as mental and emotional stress, high blood pressure, diabetes or prostate problems—or as a result of poor lifestyle choices. (Smoking, for example, has been implicated as a risk factor for erectile dysfunction. Alcohol and various illicit drugs—including Ecstasy—also increase the risk for erectile dysfunction or other sexual problems.) The good news: Jumpstarting your health won't just improve your vitality and well-being, it'll help you become a masterful lover.

Category #4
If a physical injury has impaired your sexual performance, please follow the various protocols outlined in Chapters 7 to 17, two to three times a day. This system works directly with the electrical energy that flows through your body and enables you to become erect. As you learn to activate and direct that energy, you'll be able to cultivate and apply your inner healing power. And learning to apply this healing energy includes the ability to direct it to your groin (or other injured areas), speeding up the healing process.

SEX ESSENTIALS

Being sexually aroused creates a powerful energy. Our bodies demand and need energy to function. As we learn to balance our energy and allow it to flow freely within the body, we increase our potential—our creativity, our ability to accomplish and express and achieve. By increasing and freeing the flow of our vital life force, we also intensify our sexual experience, enabling the energy of arousal to flow throughout our bodies and setting the stage for multiple waves of orgasm.

However, when our life energy isn't able to flow freely, we experience the opposite. We become blocked and explode out in the form of an ejaculation. The more energy we lose, the weaker we become. Over time, such excessive losses of energy can leave a man run down or in ill health or worse. It's important to learn how to increase your arousal energy, which—when carefully cultivated and directed—can expand your orgasmic experience as well as your appreciation of yourself as you become a long-lasting lover.

YOUR BEST SHOT

Far too often and for too long men have felt the only way they could improve their sex lives was by giving it their best shot and hoping they didn't ejaculate too soon—or by taking a pill. To slow their ejaculation, many men fall back on mathematics, imagining that if they can just concentrate on counting (or distract themselves in some other way), they may last longer and not be embarrassed by premature ejaculation.

A TIME-HONORED SYSTEM

The methods found in the *9 Steps to Building Your Sexual Stamina* training system are time-honored and part of a larger "mind/body" approach to health and wellness. The benefits of mind/body medicine have been confirmed by a substantial body of scientific research, and the approach has gained many advocates within the so-called mainstream medical community. In time, *9 Steps to*

Building Your Sexual Stamina will be heralded as a vital set of life skills for men's sexual health.

The message is important. You can have long-lasting sexual experiences and multiple orgasms without taking pills or turning to creams or herbal remedies. Sexual growth, sexual skills and sexual mastery are based on the right training—founded in discipline, awareness, energy activation, balance and harmony. Thus, a major solution to men's sexual problems involves coordinating mind and body, intent and action, through focused attention and controlled breathing. Our training system will show you the way.

To understand how to take command of your lover's body, you need to become aware of her strengths, weaknesses, likes and dislikes. In order to make a deeper connection with her body, it's essential to learn and understand the various energies that are at work within your own.

Next, you must learn to be proactive in the use of this dynamic and subtly flowing sexual energy. In order to be an effective lover, you need to be familiar with the various stages of your sexual energy. There are two main stages of energy that you'll learn to recognize and use. The first is when your sexual energy is at rest or in a non-aroused state; the second is when you're sexually aroused.

STRAIGHT TO THE POINT

By now, you probably have a number of questions, such as:

1. **What and where is my sexual muscle group?**
2. **How do I build my sexual muscle group?**
3. **And how do I use it to improve my sex life?**

YOUR SEXUAL MUSCLE GROUP

The **sexual muscle group** is more than likely a new term to most men. It refers to the group of muscles (large and small) and related structures, including the prostate gland, centering on your groin and making up the pelvic floor at the base of your torso. These muscles converge at a point between the anus and testicles for men (and between the anus and vagina for women). Think of the physical part of your body's sexual performance: That's the essence of your sexual muscle group in action.

The sexual muscle group—the prostate gland and the muscles and tendons that surround it—can be toned, trained and strengthened. This concept is pretty basic: Just as you can build your biceps, triceps, quads and overall endurance through the right exercises (weight training, aerobics, etc.), so too can you build your sexual muscle group. The key, however, is following the right training regimen.

Your sexual muscle group also encompasses several circular sets of muscles that act as shut-off valves. These circular muscles are called ring muscles and are located at the anus, the perineum and the tip of the penis. There are also sets of ring muscles at the base of the penis and connected to the bladder, as well as others that you'll learn to recognize and use as you progress in your training.

HOW TO BUILD AND STRENGTHEN YOUR SEXUAL MUSCLE GROUP

The ancient masters of lovemaking from India and China viewed the human body, the mind and emotions as a vehicle or container for energy or the life force. However, they believed that the container had holes in it. The holes mean that our life energy can leak out. When a man has an ejaculation he loses a vast amount of this energy or life force, which—as it flows out of the body—leaves the body weak.

Ejaculation does not revitalize the body. It weakens the body, mind and emotions. Sexual arousal, on the other hand, revitalizes both mind and body—and its positive emotional effects also promote healing.

Just as the penis elongates in lovemaking, it's important to learn how to extend your lovemaking skills. It's also important to remember the four ways that the penis can enter into the woman:

1. Hard
2. Firm, but slightly softer than total hardness
3. Medium hard
4. Soft

One of the keys to sexual mastery that we'll explore throughout this book is withdrawing while still erect, without ejaculation. Doing so maintains your vitality (sperm) intact and is instrumental in developing the ability to have multiple orgasms.

THE ESSENTIAL BIG THREE

There are three main sources for the energy that we need to live:

1. Air
2. Water
3. Food

SECONDARY SOURCES OF ENERGY

The body receives secondary energy through the senses:

1. Hearing
2. Vision
3. Smell
4. Taste
5. Touch

THE ESSENTIAL BIG THREE

A well-balanced sexual experience can involve all five sense organs and can affect the Essential Big Three, that is, **air, water and food:**

1. **Air.** Faster and more robust breathing patterns emerge as the sexual experience develops and excitement mounts.

2. **Water.** In the course of the sexual experience, the flow of water (in the form of blood, sexual fluids sweat and hormonal secretions) increases. The increase in blood circulation and hormone levels, in particular, helps ready the body for arousal or orgasmic release.

3. **Food.** During the sexual experience, sex is like food, and it feeds us much as real food does. But it provides its energy directly, without needing to be digested or converted. Sex arouses the appetite and can lead to cravings as well as the desire to experience and taste more.

THE SEVEN HOLES THAT RELEASE ENERGY FROM THE BODY

The human body has seven holes from which energy can escape: The five senses; the anus and the opening of the sexual organ—for men, the tip of the penis (urethra), and for women, the vaginal opening.

One of the goals of *9 Steps to Building Your Sexual Stamina* is to strengthen the various ring muscles that seal or close off the outward flow of urine and semen. Special exercises will help strengthen these muscles, allowing you to hold back the flow of your arousal and your ejaculatory fluids with ease, thereby halting the outward flow or loss of vital life force.

Learning to control and command your ejaculation starts the very first time that you are able to slow or stop this massive outpouring of energy. In doing so, you will immediately feel the effects of your energy accumulating and being redistributed throughout your body. It will revitalize your body and mind, enabling you to continue to have sex and help you achieve multiple orgasms.

EVERYONE WANTS TO ENJOY LIFE

But living (and sex) requires more than just a steady supply of energy: It also calls for balance. The more balanced and nurturing we feel, the easier it is to experience loving energy in our lives—and to share it with those around us. Learning to maintain a balance in our bodily energy enables us to experience more joy, happiness and love.

Your energy can also have a snowball effect—and you get to decide the direction in which it will flow.

- The better you feel and the more effectively you maintain or cultivate that good, joyful, loving quality, the better life becomes.

- But if you indulge your worst feelings and keep feeding the negative qualities—like anger, fear, bitterness, arrogance, etc.—the worse life becomes.

Sexual energy has a very attractive and magnetic quality because of how good it can make us feel. We seek joy in most of the things we do. But when we don't find joy in life, we are likely to experience its negative opposite—emotional pain. Our powerful attraction to sex is inextricably related to the heightened sense of energy flow that we feel in body (senses, organs and glands), mind (clarity and purpose) and emotions (joy, happiness and love).

ENERGY FLOW IS WHAT MAKES THE MALE PENIS ERECT

The ancients have referred to this energy by many names, including qi (pronounced "chee")—also written chi or ki—Prana, Kundalini, life force, Holy Spirit, love, bliss, etc. This energy flow may be experienced as tingling, electrical warmth, waves and other sensations. Some people, for example, are able to see energy as colors, patterns or visions.

Some ancient healing methods involve transforming sexual arousal into energetic awareness and directing this energy through the body. At its most advanced, this channeling of sexual energy can involve the exchange of energy with one's partner. An elevated flow of sexual energy is nurturing and healing on many levels of a person's mind, body and emotional makeup. This type of energy exchange—when cultivated together—catapults the lovers into hours and hours of sexual ecstasy and clarity.

It's important to note that I plan to offer sexual energy training methods for women. For men, *9 Steps to Building Your Sexual Stamina: The Ultimate Mind/Body System for Men* is the definitive guide to creating your bridge into better, long-lasting sex.

SHE BEGS, "PLEASE DON'T STOP!"— AND HE SIGHS, "OOPS ..."

After spending hours, days, weeks or even years of courting, dating and romancing ... to finally get the woman of your dreams in bed with you! There's great anticipation on your part and perhaps high expectations on hers. You've both wondered, teased and talked about finally sharing this loving time together. You're both aroused, eager and attracted to each other. Now's the time to make love and share this powerful moment. WAIT A MINUTE! Did I just write, "Moment"? Oh no ... And did I just write, "Wait a Minute"?

Women don't want a moment—or a minute—man, so let's **stop**! It's time for a rewrite ...

HOW LONG CAN YOU LAST?

Now it's time for you to make love. Maybe it's soft and gentle or maybe you're ready for some hot, raw, primal sex. Either way, as you go deeper into the act and relationship, you begin to share all of your passion and receive all of her deeply emotional heartfelt love. Now you both start to discover the erotic pleasures that are yours to express and experience together. It's incredible!

But how long will you last? A minute or two? Maybe 15 or 20—or, if luck's on your side, as long as half an hour. No matter, it's over much too quickly. Now your luck—and your magic—are gone, but she keeps on rocking and wiggling, and you know there's something inside of her that's still not satisfied. You, however, are done ... *finito*. Instead of taking care of business—kissing, sucking and touching her all over—you're sucking air and headed for the comatose. You're numb and empty, and now your emotions are flying. If you don't believe this ... why do you withdraw?

In the beginning of the relationship, you may have held her so tight that you'd almost crush her, so eager that you were practically tearing her clothes off. Now it may have come to the point that you don't want to talk or even be touched after you ejaculate.

YOU'RE EXHAUSTED!!!

The exhaustion is all over you. You're done; you feel empty. Why? Because you ejaculated, you shot your load long before she climaxed. Long before either of you were able to experience multiple orgasms. You hardly got started. All the vitality that your body could muster up just went out of you, and now you're chasing after sleep in order to revitalize yourself. When a man ejaculates, the ancient texts refer to the experience as a little death.

This basic scenario is played out, over and over, night after night, in most lovemaking sessions.

But it's time to become a longer-lasting lover. It's time to become sexually empowered and to develop the skills that will change your life and your sexual experiences **forever!**

TIME TO BUILD YOUR SEXUAL MUSCLE GROUP

The **bottom line** ... to be an effective lover, you must learn to improve your sexual performance. You need to sharpen your skills and take command of your sexual muscle group. Doing so is the only way you can ever become a masterful lover and last longer in bed.

If you've never studied the art of lovemaking, then you're probably operating on the basis of a limited range of personal experience with sex. Not to detract from that

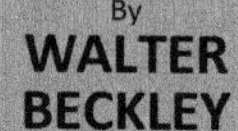

experience, but no matter how extensive, it's personal and finite: There's a lot more out there to be learned.

DON'T BE LIKE MOST MEN IN THE BEDROOM ... UNSKILLED AND UNTRAINED IN THE ART OF SEX AND LOVEMAKING

It's important to grow, not just physically, but mentally, emotionally and spiritually. And you need to expand your sexual abilities as well. When making love, it's important that you keep yourself open to learning about your body, mind, emotions, sexual energy and sexual capacity.

PARTNER MATCH-UP

Your limitations, needs and desires—your fulfillment and satisfaction—will in some cases match those of your partner. At other times, the two of you will experience friction and a sense of working at cross-purposes. Some 55% of couples pretend to accept these limitations and unfulfilled desires. They accept disappointment in order to maintain an unsatisfying relationship.

Sometimes just one partner ends up pretending to be OK with being unfulfilled, whether mentally, physically, emotionally or sexually. In far too many cases, one or both partners make a decision to sell themselves and their relationship short. They stick with the status quo in order not to be alone.

Learning to fulfill your partner in your sexual life can open new doors of communication and shared understanding.

SEXUALLY AROUSED AND UNFULFILLED

To avoid leaving your partner sexually unfulfilled, you must learn to nurture her into a deep orgasmic experience and open that space in which she feels safe, loved and important to you. This will reap vast rewards in and out of bed. She will appreciate that you put her needs before your own; again, this type of sacrifice goes a long way in any relationship.

BUILDING YOUR SEXUAL MUSCLES AND SKILLS

Why should you learn to build your sexual muscle group and improve your sexual skills? Let me ask you first another question. In your life, which would you prefer, knowing how to do something better than 98% of people or remaining ignorant and continuing to make mistakes and destroy the people and things that you care about most?

When your lover isn't being satisfied, it affects both of you and can extend well beyond the bedroom. It may affect how she relates to others, perhaps at her job or with her friends. It can affect your children, too. And she could confide in her mother, sisters, girlfriends, etc. This, of course, wouldn't reflect well on you. Thoughts like this may never cross your mind, but such things happen.

Some women love to talk, and women love to talk to each other about their feelings. You don't want your sexual skills to be on the negative side of women's conversations. And if you haven't trained, that's probably where you stand. If you find yourself wondering, when you enter the room and they're all smiling, if the joke's on you (and your shortcomings in the bedroom), you have a problem. Even if you know she really loves you, it won't matter. Most men are boys when it comes to the issue of sexual performance.

I like the United States Postal Service slogan, "**We deliver for you.**" But I really love the theme of Nike's ads: "**Just Do It.**" It's important to know how to deliver the goods each and every time you decide to "Just do it."

IMPROVING YOUR SEXUAL SKILLS

What should you focus on to improve your sexual skills? This isn't about pickup lines or what you say to charm your partner out of her clothes. It's about what comes next. *9 Steps to Building Your Sexual Stamina* is a book that will teach you how to build and take command of your sexual energy, help you last longer and use your penis more effectively and—above all—have great sex each and every time.

You'll learn to love her with confidence—to take her wholly, body, mind and emotions—to let her know the feeling of your hard, erect, relentless penis lifting her to ecstasy.

Over time, this sexual connection will increase her sexual energy and orgasmic pleasure. Once her arousal energy is built up and dammed like a river, you'll learn how to release it and carry her to orgasmic bliss. When she lets go completely, she'll be in heaven. This can last for minutes or hours. But it's something that many women have never experienced. By learning to take your woman there, you'll become her long-lasting lover and sexual hero.

But getting her to this state of sexual bliss can be as tough as getting through locked and barred palace doors. In order to gain entry, you've got to get past her guards. When she lets her guard down and opens herself to you, you'll be her hero, conqueror and lover all in one. You will have become the one, true King of her throne.

Reaching this sacred place, this orgasmic space, takes time. Three minutes—even 20 minutes—probably isn't going to suffice. But when a man has total mastery over his penis and can last for hours or even days without ejaculation during sex, her whole understanding of sexual love will be transformed.

This system is an action guide designed to teach you how to overcome and tackle your toughest sexual challenges. It will help you enrich your sexual relationship—first, through self-knowledge and then by understanding and more fully satisfying your lover.

The methods, tools and assignments in this training manual are designed to direct you and your partner into a more deeply satisfying sexual relationship. When you realize and experience sex in this way, the confidence and command that you have over yourself and your sexual energy will be empowering.

And success will build on success. You'll be catapulted into a deeper, more intimate relationship with yourself, with life and with others. Learning that you can have and maintain positive sexual relationships will deepen your confidence, and you'll find yourself better able to turn things around, not just in your sexual relationship but in all aspects of life.

As you embark on the *9 Steps to Building Your Sexual Stamina* training system, I want you to consider all of the things you'll have to learn and all the time you'll need to put into training and retraining yourself. You'll need to practice, practice, practice until you get it right. Sometimes you may drop the ball and ejaculate too soon. Old problems can be hard to escape. But feeling the power and experiencing the satisfaction you get from being able to last longer will keep you headed toward total mastery.

I've trained men from all over the world, ranging in age from 18 to 73, and I tell you this, **"if they can do it, so can**

you." You may feel discouraged at times, but just tell yourself: "If they can do it, so can I."

Once you've mastered the skills and gained a higher level of proficiency, once you've experienced and enjoyed some of the benefits, there will be no turning back. Your lover will thank you over and over again. So be patient with yourself as you learn to become sexually empowered.

But let's take things one step at a time.

2
CHALLENGES OF LIFE

Perhaps you've received a wake-up call. Maybe you lost your lover, girlfriend or wife and family. Perhaps you even lost her to another man (or woman) because of poor sexual performance, emotional disconnection or other issues. It's time to be accountable; it's time to address the issue of sexual inadequacy before it can rear its ugly head again.

WHAT WOMEN WANT: FIVE SEXUAL SECRETS

THE 1st SECRET. Women want to share themselves in this sacred act of lovemaking. And they want it as much as men do. But they also want, as Lionel Richie sings, an "endless love." If you can become a really good friend, that's a bonus, and she'll probably love you even more. But what she wants is an endless love—and a tireless lover.

THE 2nd SECRET. Women enjoy being sexed up and made love to all at the same time. She wants to feel your passion and desire for her.

THE 3rd SECRET. A woman wants someone who can take control of her body in a commanding way while still letting her feel safe. She wants a man who can transport her—who can lift her into the full experience of bliss. But she wants to feel safe as you take her sexually to her limits and beyond. Staying erect longer is one of the best ways to accomplish this.

THE 4th SECRET. In loving, women want to let go of all their worries and concerns—not just about sex but about life and all they go through. Again, this is about feeling safe.

THE 5th SECRET. A woman longs for a lover who can take her there, keep her there and fill her with waves of ecstasy and bliss that only deep, long-lasting sexual pleasure can bring.

THE 6th SECRET (THIS IS A BONUS). Most women have never experienced an energetic lover. In particular, I mean a man who can last for hours and have multiple orgasms without ejaculating. And virtually none have experienced a man capable of sending energy from his penis directly into her vagina so she feels waves of warm, electric, tingling energy flowing throughout her body.

BEYOND COMPARE

Once you've completed and learned to apply the *9 Steps to Building Your Sexual Stamina* training system, you'll feel the improvement in your sexual performance. But while mastery of these skills is important, it doesn't negate the need to achieve emotional balance.

Make sure that you take the time to visit this very important Web site:

http://www.breakthroughintogreatness.com

Register your name, e-mail or mailing address so you can receive information and training that will help you empower your masculine emotional energy so you can learn to feed the people in your life in a skilled and emotionally supportive way.

BALANCING YOUR BODY

As many people have discovered, practicing these high-level sexual training methods can leave a person feeling highly energized. And you can expect the same: Your mind, body and emotions will be revitalized and reinvigorated. At advanced levels, you'll learn how to harness and channel that energy in some very powerful and creative ways.

Some other positive notes about this training: Imagine what it would feel like to see your lover deeply satisfied after making love for hours, while you are still unspent and going strong. Yet at the same time, you fell wholly satisfied—having experienced two, three or more orgasms—as you decide when you want to let go and release that stored-up energy in a powerful ejaculation.

PRE-EJACULATION

Most men have absolutely no control; they're unable to stop or delay their ejaculation response. For most, there's no "deciding" about ejaculation. It's as unintentional and uncontrollable as an avalanche. The problem is that all too often they let go just when they should be bringing their partner to orgasm and enjoying her ride. After completing this training, you'll be able to overcome something that 99% of the sexually active men on this planet struggle with day after day—ejaculating too soon. It's time to take action to become a better and longer-lasting lover by studying the *9 Steps to Building Your Sexual Stamina*.

TRAINING | GOALS | PERFORMANCE | COMPLETION

After completing the *9 Steps to Building Your Sexual Stamina* training system, you'll have the skills to master longer erections. You'll gain even more confidence over time, as you take greater command over your penis and the muscles that can slow or stop ejaculation. Make no mistake: Your sperm is the keeper of your strength, your will and your power. It's a creative force of life. Here, for example, is an illuminating story about a famous and powerful fighter.

MIKE TYSON'S STORY

During the movie *Tyson*, a 2008 documentary, there's a point at which Tyson talks about his sexual life.

He recalls that during the early years of his boxing career, he was celibate for a solid five years. This was during the time when he reigned supreme as the undisputed heavyweight champion of the world. His punching power was clean and exacting; his body chiseled razor-sharp; his movements were quick and fast.

In contrast, when you look at the following years, when his career was on the skids, the problem wasn't simply that he had gotten out of shape and was partying too much. He was dissipating his sexual energy in about the worst way possible. As a champion, he knew better than to have sex and ejaculate just before a fight. But when he was on that losing streak, his losses marked his loss of vitality—dissipated through casual sex and ejaculating instead of holding onto his power. Certainly, Mike faced some very heavy emotional losses as well. But if he had maintained his discipline, if he had strengthened his sexual muscle group, he could have avoided that dissipation of strength. Perhaps he could have retired undefeated. A man's power, agility and health are deeply connected to his retention of his sperm.

YOUR SPERM IS LIKE LIQUID GOLD

This is groundbreaking information that every man should understand in order to live in balance: Your sperm is liquid gold. It helps manifest the health, power and vitality of your body, mind and emotions.

BECOME AN LLL (AKA LONG-LASTING LOVER)

P.S. Your lady will thank you again and again for learning to build your sexual muscle group and for becoming an LLL.

THE TRAINING

To achieve mind-blowing, world-class results—to be a Michael Jordan or Tiger Woods with the woman (or women) in your life—to perform like the undefeated world champion of the bedroom—you must learn to BUILD YOUR SEXUAL MUSCLE GROUP. Learn what you can do for yourself first in order to satisfy her over and over again.

THE GOAL

Learn to be fierce and robust in and out of the bedroom. Build a sexually energetic connection within yourself and others. Doing so will lead to deep, long-lasting and satisfying relationships in all aspects of your life.

PERFORMANCE

Don't allow concerns about sexual performance to undermine your confidence or turn your life upside-down. Don't allow the woman you love to lack for anything in your loving. It's time to change your sexual performance and be the long-lasting lover you were meant to be.

COMPLETION

No one needs to be told the difference between hot and cold. The distance between a professional and a rank amateur is immense. So, too, is that between a skilled lover and an untrained one—and, just like with hot and cold, no one has to be told the difference.

THE GENERAL PLAN FOR THIS BOOK

Chapters 1 to 6 are intended to raise your awareness about sexual issues generally.

Chapters 7 to 17 will provide step-by-step instruction and practical exercises that will show you how to strengthen your sexual muscle group.

FOR A MORE IN-DEPTH CONNECTION AND UNDERSTANDING, HEAR AND SEE OUR AUDIO AND VIDEO SERIES

When you join our Elite Membership site, you'll gain access to our audio and video library, which will enhance your learning experience. Plus, you'll get bonus information that will enable you to become a master in the art of lovemaking.

Go to:

http://www.BuildingYourSexualStamina.com/member

**IN ORDER TO BE DIFFERENT,
DO SOMETHING DIFFERENT**

**IN ORDER TO BE THE BEST LOVER YOU CAN BE,
COMPLETE THE *9 STEPS TO BUILDING YOUR SEXUAL STAMINA* TRAINING—AND
UNLEASH THE POWER WITHIN!**

TURN THE PAGE NOW TO GET STARTED!

3
SEXUAL HEALING POWER SKILLS

It's important to become familiar with the terms "yin" and "yang" and their underlying meaning. Yin and yang represent opposing forces or opposite energy polarities.

The concepts come from the ancient Chinese Taoist philosophy about the life force known as qi or chi. They are deeply rooted in Chinese approaches to health and wellness, including qigong (chi kung, chi gong), Traditional Chinese Medicine, acupuncture, tai chi, etc.

Yin is like the "–" (negative) side, say, of a battery or magnet; yang is the "+" (positive) side. They are seemingly separate and opposing forces; yet they are at the same time wholly interconnected and interdependent.

You may be wondering, "So what does all this have to do with better sex?" Simply put: When you learn how to keep your battery charged and circulate this sexual energy through your body, you last longer. If too much energy goes through an electrical circuit, you'll blow a fuse. If too much sexual energy flows into the prostate, testicles and penis, you'll also blow a fuse (ejaculate). If you can learn to disperse that energy to other parts of your body, your circuits won't overheat—you'll just keep going and going and going ...

Yin and yang represent the “unity in opposites,” a principle that can be observed all around us—and especially in the natural world—for example, in day and night, life and death, and male and female. Simply put, Yin and Yang can be interpreted and defined as “female” and “male” or as “negative” and “positive." Yin and yang describe the endless pairs of opposites that we observe throughout creation.

Yin and yang are based on the polarity of the energy, electricity, qi or life force that flows within everything, both living and inanimate.

CHART OF OPPISITES:

YIN	YANG
Female	Male
Negative	Positive
Stillness	Action
Space	Object
Black	White
Cold	Hot
Water	Fire
Hatred	Love
Etc.	Etc.

Yin and yang relationships are pairs of opposites. Yin gives rise to yang, and yang gives rise to yin. In essence, each unfolds and produces the other, much like night (yin) follows day (yang) and day follows night ... Yin and yang are constantly at work. This is the natural order of things in life.

So you see, it's natural for men and women to be attracted to one another. Both feel (and know) something within—that they are mutual counterparts, with each part finding its true completion in joining the other. Men and women can be energetically aroused—drawn or repelled through thoughts, emotions, physical attraction, smells, taste, sound and touch. We often say that a particularly charismatic person has a "magnetic personality," but the truth is that energy—magnetic or electric or whatever you want to call it—characterizes all of us.

When our life force takes the particular form of sexual energy, the mutual attraction or connection is at its most explosive. Sexual energy is the only energy that can be multiplied not just to sustain life but to **new** life.

But sex is complicated: Our sexual desires can be both creative and destructive. Sexual energy can be used in very erotic and creative ways or in negative ways that cause pain and fear.

YIN AND YANG AND SEX

The penis can experience a multitude of changes. When flaccid and unaroused, the penis is in a yin or negative state. Its energy charge is negative, and it's withdrawn and in a state of stillness.

When aroused, the penis enters a state of yang or positive energy—its state is positive, and it's erect and ready for action.

These two states are total opposites; however, there are thousands of incremental variations—a sliding scale that runs between the extremes hard and soft.

WHAT HAPPENS WHEN A MAN WANTS TO HAVE SEX WITH A WOMAN WHEN HIS PENIS IS SOFT OR YIN?

If the desire to have sex is there but the penis is still "sleeping"—that is, in a soft, "yin" state—there are several possible explanations for what's preventing the flow of positive, yang energy into the penis.

1. Physical damage to the penis, the nervous system, the brain or other organs or glands.
2. Sickness, bad health, diabetes, high blood pressure, etc.
3. Drugs, alcohol, etc.

4. Prescription medications.
5. Emotional imbalance: anxiety, stress, fear, worry, etc.

If you are working through physical damage to your body that has affected your penis yang energy (as outlined in point 1), this book will give you some insight into various ways to stimulate the flow of yang and overcome the effects of yin energy into your penis.

YOUR EMOTIONS CAN STOP YOUR ERECTION

Your emotions play such a vital role in your sexual ability and performance that they can make or break you. When you understand the power of these feelings, you'll never find yourself in a position of wanting to make love but finding yourself unable to do so.

When you find the balance between your yin and yang, your negative and positive feelings, you enter a higher level of awareness—and power—in your sexual relationships. By learning to move with ease between yin and yang, softness and hardness, you will begin to master your erections. For further discussion of the role of clarity and the importance of balance in your emotions, visit:

http://www.breakthroughintogreatness.com

SIX KEY POINTS ON THE PATH TO DEVELOPING YOUR SEXUAL POWER

1. Stay open to learning more about your anatomy and sexual strengths and weaknesses.

2. Learn to recognize the qi energy or life force in your body. (This is easy: qi energy becomes bioelectrical in your body, and it is this positive bioelectrical energy that makes you erect.)

3. Learn to cultivate this energy so that it grows and strengthens your mind, body and emotions.

4. Learn to move or circulate the qi energy so that it flows into the right channels, organs and glands in a consistent and harmoniously balanced way. These (and the following points) are the skills that you'll be learning in Chapters 7 to 17 of this book.

5. Learn to receive and draw energy into your body.

6. Learn to transfer this energy to another person. Again, these are skills that you'll be learning in Chapters 7 to 17 of this book.

As you begin to develop your sexual muscle group, you'll start to experience more enriching aspects of yourself and your partner. Over time, your relationship will deepen and become stronger and more nurturing. The result: You will be able to **grow** through life and not just **go** through life. When we learn to channel the electric potential of our sexual experiences, we will nourish ourselves as well as our partners. This, in turn, can enhance our creativity and self-worth, which increases our value in the world. You will find that the benefits extend across all your relationships as you become more **inwardly centered, powerful** and **energized**.

The power that lies in our sexual energy can create life and—when harnessed effectively—can strengthen our health, our minds and our careers, relationships, emotions and finances—as well as the spiritual and energy-centered aspects of our existence.

UNDERSTANDING THE FEMALE OR YIN ENERGY

A woman's sexual energy or power is sometimes regarded as being like ice. But like most generalizations, this one falls well short of the truth. Some women are less interested in sex—some may almost reject it outright. But others are as fiery as the midday sun. Likewise, some women take time before they are open to it, while others are easily aroused and may crave sexual contact as much (or even more) than you. And, of course, most women fall somewhere between these extremes.

Given this wide range of sexual responses, a man should study and persevere until he finds his match. If you are married or have a partner whose sexual interest just doesn't seem well-matched to your own but you truly love her, don't worry, there's still hope. As her lover, you can learn to release her from the fears or pains—physical, mental or emotional—that impede the full expression of her sexual energies.

However, doing so will take time, patience and a strong commitment on your part to helping her unfold into her true orgasmic ecstasy and power. Only when **you** become **highly skilled in the art of the bedroom** and **the art of lovemaking,** will you be able to accompany her into the pleasures of being a woman. Your abilities as a long-lasting lover will be vital in her rebirth into the power of love, joy and ecstasy. But first you must get yourself together; only then—and, of course, only when **she's** ready—will you be able to assist her.

MAKE SURE SHE FEELS SAFE

When a woman relaxes, you know she feels comfortable and safe. I repeat: When a woman feels safe, she starts to feel even more comfortable. What this means for you is that she feels more open, trusting and willing to please you—as well as to be pleased. These feelings of comfort enable her to enter into her own natural rhythm and flow.

As you learn these methods you'll turn your partner into a river of boiling sexual energy. This is highly beneficial for you.

COMMUNICATE WITH HER

Please Note: This book does not cover what to say or how to communicate with your partner in order for her to want you to make love to her. We assume that she wants you. … So let's start with your touch.

Your warm touch is your first physical contact. Your warm and gentle touch will relax and communicate directly with her body, which will begin thawing her emotions. A warm and loving touch can put her mind at ease and can charge deeper circuits throughout her body. Your touch, however, should be a physical extension of her sense of safety. Slow and careful to start with, confident and in charge, yet gentle—you need to assure her that everything is all right.

When your touch brings about a sense of well-being, it will melt away any fears and misgivings. And it can cause a flow of her waters, making her vagina wet, building her arousal, her eagerness and her interest in you.

MAGNETISM = ATTRACTION

When a man can control his ejaculations, his electrical potential and magnetism increases, and his penis goes from being a garden hose suitable for running the sprinkler to a fire hose, hard, thick and capable of keeping her safe even as her fires rage. The result, for both of you, will be exquisite states of ecstasy, bliss and pleasure. These states become more readily available to the man as he learns to draw energy from his partner through his penis into his nervous system, organs and glands in order to nourish his body. His partner can also draw energy from him in the same way.

As you become conscious of the life energy that powers lovemaking, you and your partner will find that your relationship benefits, becoming more energetic and magnetic and physical. In the process, your bodies will be reacting to the energetic forces that flow within and between you. With your electrical life energy removed, your body is little more than a piece of wood. Energy is the source of movement, change and animation. That's the reason it's so important for a man to learn to operate from the source of energy and cultivate his energetic life force—only then can he experience the highest and best use of all of his powers including his sexual healing power.

LEARNING TO BUILD YOUR SEXUAL MUSCLE GROUP

As you build your sexual muscle group, you'll learn how to:

1. Create and keep a rock-hard erection.

2. Become multi-orgasmic and not lose your erection.

3. Have long-lasting sexual encounters without taking a pill.

4. Avoid premature ejaculation.

5. Create sexual power, harmony and balance.

6. Improve your sexual communication skills.

7. Experience deeper levels of orgasm.

8. Satisfy your partner beyond orgasm.

9. Energize your testicles and improve your vitality.

10. Increase the intimacy between you and your lover.

FOR A MORE IN-DEPTH CONNECTION AND UNDERSTANDING, HEAR AND SEE OUR AUDIO AND VIDEO SERIES

When you join our Elite Membership site, you'll gain access to our audio and video library, which will enhance your learning experience. Plus, you'll get bonus information that will enable you to become a master in the art of lovemaking.

Go to:

http://www.BuildingYourSexualStamina.com/member

4
THE ART OF BEING A MULTI-ORGASMIC MAN

Being a multi-orgasmic man means being able to achieve your full orgasmic potential. When you learn to build your sexual muscle group, you will take command over your penis. It's very important for men to develop lovemaking skills that enable them to prolong sex at will, control their ejaculations, have multiple orgasms, satisfy their partners and decide when they are ready to incorporate ejaculatory release into the lovemaking session.

The multi-orgasmic man is able to broaden his sexual experience with each encounter. When you become a multi-orgasmic lover, you can make love longer (literally for hours on end). As you experience the intensity of having multiple orgasms yet maintaining control over your sexual organ and body, you'll be able to make love with a woman and have **real** confidence. Longer lovemaking sessions can bring women to full satisfaction—a deeper, more fulfilling and extended state of pleasure far beyond the normal state of orgasm.

Once you learn to experience the power and bliss of a non-ejaculatory orgasm, you'll wonder why no one had ever taught you these invaluable tools.

Being a multi-orgasmic man doesn't mean that you can't experience external ejaculation. It just means that now you have a choice. You decide how long you want to make love. You have the confidence to handle any woman (with no more need for counting or other ploys to stop yourself from ejaculating too soon). When you build your sexual muscle group there will be no need for pills or any other external assistance.

WHAT HAPPENS WHEN I EJACULATE?

Most men have no idea of what happens when they ejaculate, other than that it feels great. But to become sexually masterful, it's essential that you understand what happens in your body as you have an ejaculation. So let's take a closer look at the steps involved.

MALE EJACULATION SEQUENCE

While being stimulated—whether by yourself or by a partner whether you're dreaming about being with some lucky lady or just grinding away in your sleep—there is a sequence of well-studied events that occur as your body experiences an ejaculation. It involves four distinct phases. (See "Male Ejaculation Chart," below.):

I. Excitement Phase
II. Plateau Phase
III. Orgasm Phase
IV. Resolution Phase

Male Ejaculation Chart

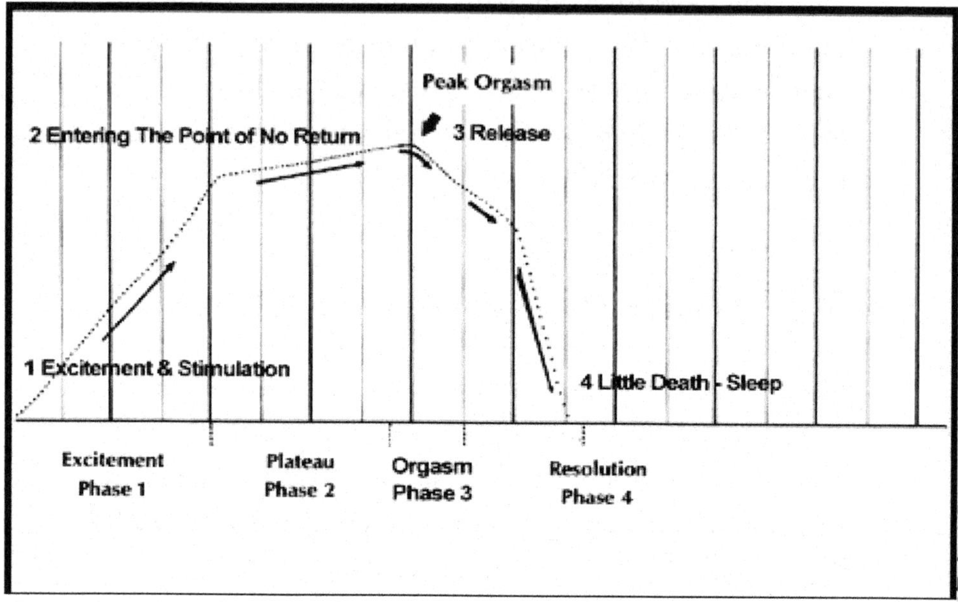

This chart shows (left to right) the pre- and post-ejaculation phases, as follows: Excitement, Plateau, Orgasm and Resolution.

Phase 1—Excitement and Stimulation

The excitement phase involves sexual stimulation. Sexual stimulation, whether physical (touch), mental (through sexual thoughts, pictures or videos) or even while asleep and having sexual dreams, can produce vasocongestion.

In vasocongestion, there's an increase in the flow of blood into the penis. Through the action of the ring muscles, this extra blood stays in the penis, resulting in an erection.

Vasocongestion can vary from one man to another. And, for a given man, it can also vary over time and due to specific circumstances.

Physical Changes During Vasocongestion

During the excitement phase a man may notice changes in the length, size, girth, hardness and sensitivity of his penis. The scrotum and testes may rise up or pull closer towards the body while the testes may even swell and increase in size. This can vary from man to man; however, many men experience a heightened sensitivity around the penis, inner thighs, nipples and other areas of the body.

Breathing patterns typically become more erratic, and blood pressure and heart rate increase. Many men experience a clenching and or tensing of various muscles. There are many visual as well as other subtle bodily changes.

Phase 2—Plateau—Entering the Point of No Return

Continued sexual stimulation results in a shift from the initial excitement phase to the second, plateau phase. The duration of the plateau phase can be either short or long and is followed by orgasm.

For many men, unfortunately, the plateau is very short. But by building your sexual muscle group, you can learn how to extend and control it.

Some Physical Changes That May Occur

As more blood flows into the penis and less flows out, the result is a firmer, harder erection. At the same time, the head of the penis expands in size as it becomes filled with blood.

One potential byproduct of sexual stimulation is a clear fluid, known as pre-ejaculate fluid, which is secreted by the Cowper's gland and helps prepare the urethra (the tube located in the penis that carries urine and semen out of the body) for the release of semen.

As a man becomes more aroused and stimulated, his testicles tend to swell and increase in size. The testes also move closer towards the body.

With continued stimulation of the penis, a deeper sense of excitement spreads throughout the body. Breathing, heart rate and blood pressure all increase further, as does the locking or tensing of muscles.

Phase 3—Orgasm—Release

The body is now ready to experience the three stages of orgasm.

The First Stage:

Once you have reached a high state of arousal, contractions will begin—specifically, in the vas deferens (or ductus deferens), the seminal vesicles and the prostate gland. (See illustration, page 78.) These actions cause seminal fluid or ejaculate to begin gathering or collecting in a pool at the base of the penis, within the prostate and urethra.

Some men describe this gathering of fluids in terms of a vibrating, tickling or pulsating sensation.

The Second Stage:
Muscle contractions increase and begin to occur in a throbbing manner at the prostate and around the urethra.

The Third Stage:
The prostate is now ready to propel or ejaculate the gathered semen through the urethra and out of the body. This release of fluids is the ejaculation and release.

Separating Orgasm from Ejaculation
For men, the excitement and stimulation phase (Phase 1) is good. And so is the plateau (Phase 2). But ejaculation (Phase 3) is more complicated. Certainly, it feels good: The contractions of orgasm (which occur at different speeds) are what men experience as the most pleasurable sensations connected with sex. On the other hand, ejaculation halts lovemaking and robs the body of vitality. The solution, the secret doorway that leads to sexual freedom for men, lies between Phase 2 and Phase 3.

Phase 4—Resolution—Recovery, Rest or Sleep

The Resolution phase refers to the period immediately following ejaculation. Resolution is when the body begins to recover and return to its "normal" state.

In short, when you have sex with ejaculation, your body enters into a recovery mode to replenish the lost fluids, energy, minerals and vitamins.

Other changes: The penis returns to its normal, flaccid state as the blood and vital energy disperse. The scrotum and testes drop down and away from the body and return to their normal size. Most men experience a general feeling of peace and relaxation.

For a time following ejaculation, a man will be physically incapable of achieving another erection. This experience is called the refractory period. It can vary in time from a few minutes to hours or—for some—even days. This refractory period generally lengthens with age; it's also longer in men who are sick, who have chronic conditions or whose health is otherwise compromised.

But when you have sex with multiple orgasms without ejaculation your body retains a heightened or energized state. For multi-orgasmic men, the refractory period is nonexistent.

ANCIENT MASTERS VERSUS THE DEFEATED WARRIOR METHOD

The ancient masters understood how to control and command their life energy, recognizing that after a man ejaculates, exhaustion and sleep take over. The ancient masters likened this sleep after ejaculation to a weakened or defeated warrior ... one left for dead. And they thought of ejaculation as a little death.

BENEFITS OF BEING A MULTI-ORGASMIC MAN

When a man becomes multi-orgasmic, he's able to have non-ejaculatory orgasms. He still experiences sensations that are similar to an ejaculation, e.g., the contractions or flutters that take place within the prostate, but he won't release any ejaculatory fluids. He will be able to keep his vital energy, allowing him to continue having sex and to experience multiple orgasms, which can become more and more intense.

Anyone can experience hours of sexual enjoyment and prolonged, multiple orgasms by building his or her sexual muscle group and learning to channel the body's inner energy.

As you learn to take command of your sexual muscle group, you will still experience Phase 1, the sexual excitement phase. (See chart, below.)

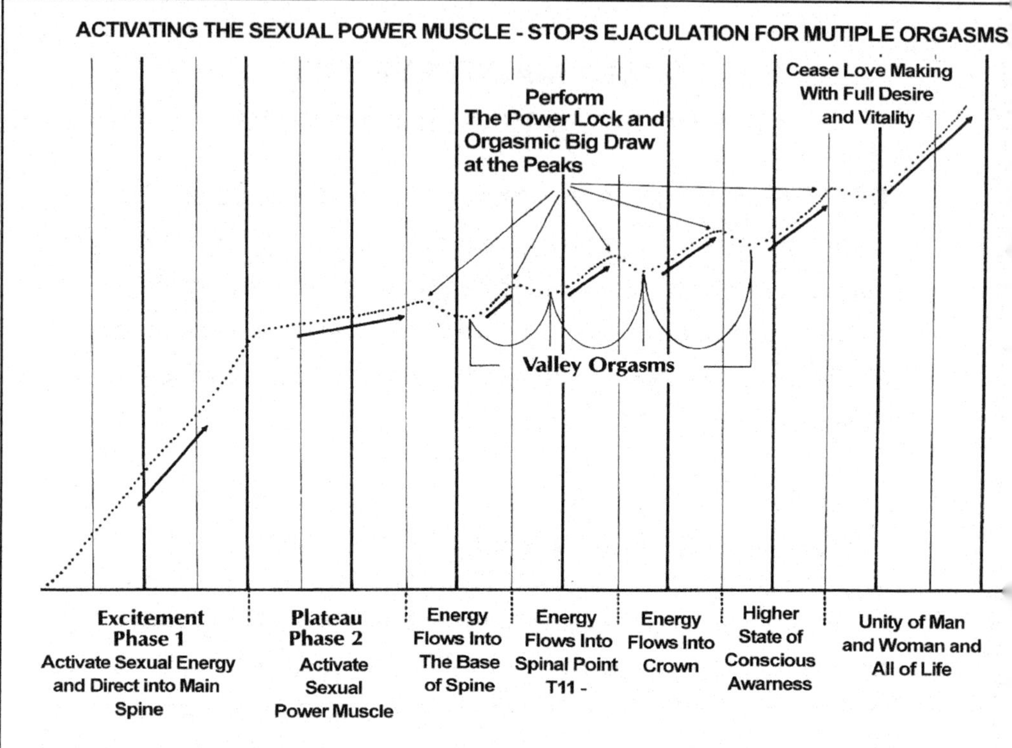

You'll also experience Phase 2, the Plateau. (See chart, above.) However, you won't enter the point of no return or ejaculate, that is, Phase 3.

As noted above, when you develop your multi-orgasmic potential, Phase 3 (ejaculation) will be eliminated. Instead, you'll divert or channel your sexual energy. You'll feel the intensity of an orgasm, but instead of that being the endpoint; you'll be able to repeat the experience over and over again. (See chart, above.)

When experiencing multiple orgasms in this way, you will ultimately enter Phase 4, the Resolution. But you'll do so on **your** terms and in a very different way from what's generally expected of that phase. By eliminating the "little death" experience, you and your partner will achieve a deep—and shared—sense of completion. Instead of feeling drained, spent, or exhausted, your mind and body will be charged with pleasure, vitality, clarity and energy. (See chart, above.)

FOR A MORE IN-DEPTH CONNECTION AND UNDERSTANDING, HEAR AND SEE OUR AUDIO AND VIDEO SERIES

When you join our Elite Membership site, you'll gain access to our audio and video library, which will enhance your learning experience. Plus, you'll get bonus information that will enable you to become a master in the art of lovemaking.

Go to:

http://www.BuildingYourSexualStamina.com/member

5
THE FORMULA FOR SURVIVING THE LITTLE DEATH (AKA EJACULATION)

According to the ancient Taoist masters of qi or life energy, ejaculation for a man is like a little death. Every time he ejaculates, it's as if he dies a little. Whether through masturbation or sexual intercourse, whether for play or procreation, when a man ejaculates, his body gathers its best nutrients and bioelectrical energy to jumpstart a new life. In so doing, the man experiences a great loss of energy. Over time, this "little death" robs a man of his vital qi, the life force or bioelectrical energy, leaving him weakened susceptible to sickness, illness and disease.

To combat this loss of energy, ancient Chinese healers and teachers established a regimen that would help men keep more of their much-needed vitality. The regimen involves learning to limit the frequency of ejaculations. By doing so, over a period of time (and depending on the man's age), he'll be able to slow the loss of energy that results from ejaculating too often.

When men find themselves in a state of diminished vitality, struggling with premature ejaculation, erectile dysfunction, physical illness, etc., it's best to limit or avoid ejaculation. It's important during such difficulties that men learn to become orgasmic, but not actually ejaculate. However, if you find that your need is so great that abstinence is impractical, you can apply this simple formula to assist you in regaining your lost vitality while also learning to overcome sickness, weakness, illness and disease.

THE FORMULA

In *The Tao of Sexology: The Book of Infinite Wisdom*, Dr. Stephen T. Chang offers the following formula for ejaculation frequency:

Age ____ x .2 = Frequency (i.e., the appropriate number of days that should pass between ejaculations).

Thus, for example:

42 (age) x .2 = 8.4

In other words, a 42-year-old man shouldn't ejaculate more frequently than once every 8.4 days.

Ejaculating with greater frequency than your age-calculated limit could lead to weakness, impotence, sexual dysfunction, sickness or even premature death.

Remember, not ejaculating is the best!

Learning to avoid ejaculation during sex or masturbation will help you maintain your vitality, which can be used to nourish and heal the body.

MODIFYING SEXUAL BEHAVIOR PATTERNS

In order to master your sexual powers, you'll need to modify certain behaviors and develop a new sense of discipline. Whether you are healthy or are sick and have sexual challenges, follow the complete *9 Steps to Building Your Sexual Stamina* system, and join our online membership program today.

To fully engage your sexual power it's important to approach your body in a nourishing manner. Thus, *9 Steps to Building Your Sexual Stamina* emphasizes not just energy flows but also sensitivity. Being too strict, hard or tough on yourself will interfere with the growth of your sexual power.

In order to make the most of your training, try keeping notes or journal your thoughts and feelings about having sex without ejaculating. The choice is between releasing energy (ejaculation) and gathering energy (orgasms).

THE NON-EJACULATION FAST

To become a master lover, you'll need to develop inner discipline. And perhaps the best test of that discipline is undertaking a non-ejaculation fast. The good news is that you don't have to give up sex. Rather, the goal is to give up ejaculation. Try doing so for five or 10 days—or even longer. It's not easy, but it'll help increase your vitality and let you test your ability to control your desires.

As you increase your non-ejaculating days, you'll increase your overall vitality as well. However, the requisite number of days will vary from man to man. So turn to the lessons and protocols outlined in Chapters 7 to 17, and start with a simple five-day non-ejaculation fast as you practice these exercises. When you start to feel more vitality, you can increase the number of days of your non-ejaculatory fast.

6
THE MALE REPRODUCTIVE SYSTEM

The male reproductive organs, or genitals, are located both inside and outside the pelvis. The male genitals include:

1. The penis
2. The testicles
3. The duct system, which is made up of the vas deferens and the epididymis
4. Cowper's gland
5. The accessory glands, which include the seminal vesicles and prostate gland (Sperm Palace)

The main part of the penis is the shaft. The tip or head of the penis, known as the glans, is extremely sensitive. And at the end of the glans is the urethral opening, which is a small slit where urine and semen exit the body. The penis is made of a spongy tissue that, when stimulated, expands and fills with blood, resulting in an erection.

When a man reaches sexual maturity, his testicles or testes can produce and store millions of sperm cells. The testicles are somewhat oval-shaped, about 2 inches long and an inch in diameter. Beside sperm, the testicles produce the hormone testosterone. Testosterone is what gives men deeper voices, bigger muscles and facial and body hair—it's also what stimulates sperm production.

Attached to the testicles are the vas deferens (or ductus deferens) and epididymis duct system, which transport the sperm.

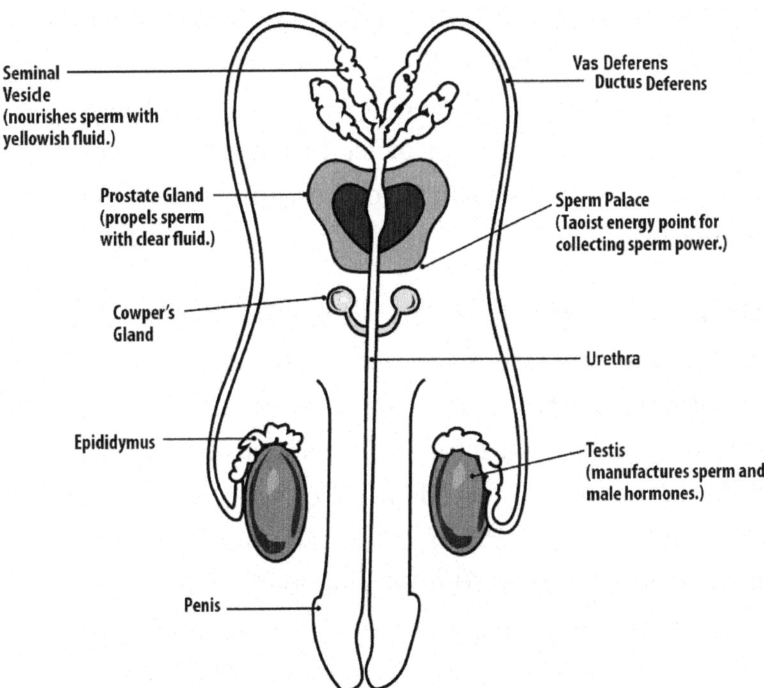

The epididymis is a set of tightly coiled tubes attached to each testicle; it collects the sperm and stores them as they mature. The vas deferens is a muscular tube that runs from the epididymis to the urethra, and the urethra, in turn, is the tube that runs the length of the penis and—during ejaculation—carries the sperm out of the body.

The scrotum is the bag or pouch-like structure located outside of the pelvis and under the penis. The epididymis and the testicles hang inside the scrotum. In order for the testicles to produce sperm, they must be kept cooler than normal body temperature. The scrotum helps to regulate the testicular temperature. When the temperature and the testicles are too cool, the scrotum will shrink or tighten, drawing the testicles closer to the body. When the testicles are too warm, the scrotum relaxes and becomes looser, so the testicles aren't as close to the body core, allowing freer circulation of air to get rid of excess heat. The signal for these changes comes from the brain and the nervous system.

The accessory glands, which include the seminal vesicles as well as the prostate gland, lubricate the duct system and provide fluids that nourish the sperm. The seminal vesicles, sac-like structures that are attached to the vas deferens and connected to the side of the bladder, contribute about 60% of the total volume of the semen (the fluid released during ejaculation, which contains the sperm); the prostate gland provides most of the rest.

The prostate surrounds the ejaculatory ducts at the base of the urethra just below the bladder.

As noted above, the urethra is the tube that passes through the penis and carries the semen out of the body. It's also the channel through which urine passes or exits the body.

THE SEQUENCE OF EJACULATION

1. The testicles produce millions of sperm cells each and every day.

2. The sperm then collect in the epididymis, where they mature.

3. Then they enter the vas deferens, or sperm duct.

4. The seminal vesicles and prostate gland produce a whitish fluid called seminal fluid.

5. When a man is sexually stimulated, the seminal fluid mixes with sperm from the testicles to form semen.

6. The penis, which is usually soft and flaccid, becomes erect or hard when sexually stimulated or excited, as blood fills its spongy tissues—the result, when sustained, is an erection.

7. The stiff erect penis is inserted into the female's vagina.

8. As a result of penile stimulation, muscles around the reproductive organs, mainly the perineum muscles, start to contract and force semen through the duct system and urethra.

9. Semen is ejected out of the man's body through his urethra—the process termed **ejaculation**.

Each time a man ejaculates, he can release as many as 500 million sperm. This entails a significant diminution of his energy supply. A man's body doesn't know the difference between having sex for fun or for creating another life. It treats each sexual episode as if it were about to create life, committing all the best substances available in the body to that act of creation. When a man ejaculates, he releases a tremendous amount of sperm, which contain the vital life force, that is, the electrical or magnetic energy needed to jumpstart the female egg and create new life.

THE NEXT STAGE

Congratulation, you are to be commended for having completed the first phase of this book. You are now ready to begin your training.

FOR A MORE IN-DEPTH CONNECTION AND UNDERSTANDING, HEAR AND SEE OUR AUDIO AND VIDEO SERIES

When you join our Elite Membership site, you'll gain access to our audio and video library, which will enhance your learning experience. Plus, you'll get bonus information that will enable you to become a master in the art of lovemaking.

Go to:

http://www.BuildingYourSexualStamina.com/member

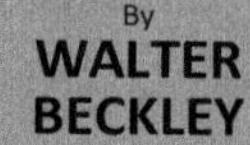

9 STEPS TO THE BEST SEX EVER

YOUR PERSONAL TRAINING BEGINS HERE

Chapters 7–17

7
STEP 1—SEX AND BREATHING

PART 1—THE FOCUSED-POWER BREATHING METHOD

At first, this part of the training program may seem hard to connect with the goal of sexual mastery, but I promise you, when you learn to activate the power within your body through the Focused-Power Breathing Method®, you will understand the connection. This part of the training teaches you how you can make love with power and ease when you learn to harness your breath. When you learn the Focused-Power Breathing Method®, you'll gain the ability to calm your body before you become prematurely excited.

The Focused-Power Breathing Method®, at its highest level, becomes orgasmic breathing or blissful breathing. It's important to understand that there is unlimited power in the air that moves in and out of your body and that you are about to learn how to connect with this power.

WATCHING YOUR BODY BREATHE

You might be wondering why Focused-Power Breathing is so important for your sexual strength.

The next time you have a sexual encounter, watch and count the variations in your breathing—and just how irregular it becomes. Pay attention to the number of times your breathing changes from soft to hard, fast to slow, shallow to deep, long to short and how often you stop or hold your breath before exhaling. You'll notice that you have little or no control over your breathing, particularly as you get closer and closer to ejaculating.

As you learn to breathe the Focused-Power Breathing way, you'll learn to relax and become wakefully alert at the same time. As you learn to watch and be in command of your breathing, you'll be amazed at how important your breathing patterns are—in regulating your sexual energy and in controlling your bodily functions.

THE IMPORTANCE OF THE BREATH

Think about it: If your breath were to stop flowing in and out of your body, first, you'd go unconscious—you'd pass out—then you'd die. It would only take a few minutes. On the other hand, the more energy you draw into your body, the stronger you become.

We've all seen, heard or read about how the old frail master throws the young muscle-bound man around with ease or how a mother can lift a car off her child. The master has trained his body for years and can consistently connect with the inner source of power and use it at will. While the mother because of great determination, love and willpower, can connect with the inner source of her power and lift the car. I hope that these illustrations drive home the importance of training your breath verses waiting for your power to miraculously turn on because you're about to ejaculate. You must learn to activate, cultivate and circulate this inner connection—and that's what Focused-Power Breathing will give your body and your life—sexual vitality and overall well-being.

There is hidden power within your breath. There are thousands upon thousands of writings throughout history attesting to the power of the breath.

The Focused-Power Breathing Method® is designed to help you access and release your inner source of power. Within your body, that inner source of power manifests itself as bioelectrical energy. Your inner source of power is easily accessed through breathing.

When you learn what Focused-Power Breathing can teach you about breathing, you'll become more conscious, alert and energized. You'll have a real sense of inner power. The ancient Chinese healing and martial arts systems—including acupuncture, tai chi and qigong (chi kung)—all work by recognizing and cultivating qi, the life force or bioelectrical energy. This energy flows through the body's meridian system. In much the same way as veins carry blood, the meridians carry electrical energy throughout the body. And modern imaging technologies—including electroencephalograms (EEGs), positron emission tomography (PET) and functional magnetic resonance imaging (fMRI)—have been used in the study of qi-based practices, such as acupuncture and meditation.

In China, qigong (or chi kung) is an ancient art. Loosely translated, it means “breathing energy exercise.” Once again, the term “qi” (or chi) refers to the vital energy or life force. “Gong” (or “kung”) means discipline or exercise. Their combination describes the practice of evoking and channeling the body’s life force, its bioelectrical energy.

In particular, qigong refers to a meditative practice that features controlled breathing and slow, graceful movements designed to strengthen an individual’s qi.

Masters and serious practitioners of qigong are known for some amazing feats. For example, at one level, a student of qigong can achieve what’s known as an “Iron Crotch.” Individuals who do so can easily withstand powerful blows—not simply to the body but directly to the groin—without discomfort. How can that be possible? They do so by using their minds, controlled breathing and coordinated movements to redirect their vital qi to protect various parts of the body as needed.

Imagine how your partner will feel when you’re able to move your breath and qi into your penis, not only making it rock solid—hard as steel—but also being able to last for hours without experiencing a sudden loss of power.

THE FOCUSED-POWER BREATHING METHOD®

Life starts and ends with your breath. The quality of your life is the direct product of how and how well you breathe.

Focused-Power Breathing reestablishes the depth, the energetic quality and the joy in your breathing. Focused-Power Breathing directly enhances the quality of your daily life and your sexual vitality. It also contributes to greater longevity and strength.

However, in order to breathe correctly and be able to direct your breath throughout your body, you must **practice** and master each lesson without skipping ahead or moving on to the next lesson.

As you practice the Focused-Power Breathing Method® you will naturally draw more blood into the capillaries of your penis (and throughout your body). Your blood vessels will open and expand, letting more blood into your penis in a natural way. Breathing in this way is a natural alternative to Viagra.

Through Focused-Power Breathing, you will consciously activate—and integrate your awareness of—the inner source of power in your body and life. This inner source of power is like a battery with an endless supply of energy. The benefits of this exercise include:

1. Deep oxygenation of the body as a whole.

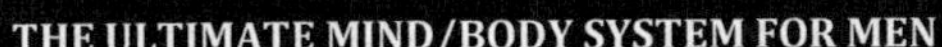

2. Healthful massage of the abdominal area, its organs and glands, through the abdominal movements associated with this form of deep breathing.

3. Better distribution of blood and energy throughout the body by the deep, diaphragm-based breathing, which acts like an energy pump.

4. Increased focus as the mind concentrates on the flow of energy through the body.

5. Heightened muscle development and overall strengthening.

Focused-Power Breathing is an exercise discipline that can help develop and define your muscles, tendons and ligaments. It also aids in grounding the life energy associated with breathing and sexual stimulation.

The exercises of Focused-Power Breathing are designed to provide a simple but highly effective way to awaken and unite body, mind and spirit—based on energy flow.

LESSON 1
FOCUSED-POWER BREATHING METHOD®
INSTRUCTIONS

1. Sit up straight.
2. Place your feet flat against the floor.
3. Set your hands over your navel, or rest them on your thighs with palms facing up.
4. Inhale (for a count of 4 or 5 seconds)—as you count and inhale, your navel area should expand.
5. Exhale (for a count of 4 or 5 seconds)—and as you count and exhale, your navel area should contract in towards your spine.
6. Breathe only through your nose.
7. Close your eyes.
8. Be very gentle.
9. Repeat this sequence for about five minutes.

Practice Focused-Power Breathing twice a day: First thing in the morning and, in the evening, an hour before or after dinner.

The Focused-Power Breathing Method® is a high-level training system. The first level of Focused-Power Breathing involves a music CD that enables you to connect with and start to feel the rhythm of your breath and energy. When your breath and inner source of power become united, the inner fire ignites. Inside the fire, you will sense a vibration that feels like joy. Some people also report a warm or tingling quality. Find this inner joy, and lose yourself in it. If you don't have the Focused-Power Breathing CD and DVD package, I highly recommend adding them to your daily practice.

To purchase the DVD and CD combination and gain a fuller mastery over your breath, visit:

http://www.BuildingYourSexualStamina.com/member

Remember to **practice** in order to advance your sexual skills!—Walter

Proceed to Chapter 8 and the next lesson.

FOR A MORE IN-DEPTH CONNECTION AND UNDERSTANDING, HEAR AND SEE OUR AUDIO AND VIDEO SERIES

When you join our Elite Membership site, you'll gain access to our audio and video library, which will enhance your learning experience. Plus, you'll get bonus information that will enable you to become a master in the art of lovemaking.

Go to:

http://www.BuildingYourSexualStamina.com/member

8
STEP 1—SEX AND BREATHING

PART 2—THE REVERSE FOCUSED-POWER BREATHING METHOD®

Congratulations, you have just completed part 1 of the Focused-Power Breathing Method®. In part 1, you learned to relax and connect with your breath in a more meditative and energetically connected way. Now that you can feel the power, in part 2, you'll learn how to breathe the energy deeper into your power center by reversing the direction of the abdominal area as you inhale and exhale.

Usually, when people inhale, their abdominal area expands out, and when they exhale the abdomen contracts. **With Reverse Focused-Power Breathing, as you inhale, your abdominal area contracts, and as you exhale, your abdominal area expands.**

Breathing in this manner offers many benefits: It improves coordination, increases abdominal strength, aids digestion. It also draws oxygen more deeply into the body. And the result of these changes is a feeling of relaxed calm, increased energy and greater control over one's sexual energy.

In the ancient Chinese and Indian disciplines, one of the primary functions of breathing exercises is to gather and store qi within the body, particularly by balancing and reversing the respiratory process. The more effective you are at controlled, dynamic breathing, the more command you will have over your basic qi energy—and your faster-moving sexual energy.

But before you can effectively handle your sexual energy, you need to start with qi, the base energy that lies behind your sexual energy.

REVERSE BREATHING METHOD

1. Sit up straight.
2. Set your feet flat against the floor.
3. Place your hands over your navel or rest them on your thighs with your palms facing up.
4. Inhale (for a count of 4 or 5 seconds), and as you inhale and count, your navel area should contract in toward your spine.
5. Exhale (for a count of 4 or 5 seconds), and as you exhale and count, your navel area should expand out.
6. Breathe only through your nose.
7. Close your eyes.
8. Be very gentle.
9. Repeat this for about 5 minutes straight.

FOR A MORE IN-DEPTH CONNECTION AND UNDERSTANDING, HEAR AND SEE OUR AUDIO AND VIDEO SERIES

When you join our Elite Membership site, you'll gain access to our audio and video library, which will enhance your learning experience. Plus, you'll get bonus information that will enable you to become a master in the art of lovemaking.

Go to:

http://www.BuildingYourSexualStamina.com/member

Take your time and learn to feel the energy in your lower belly.—*Walter*

9
STEP 2—KIDNEY ACTIVATION MASSAGE

According to Chinese medicine, the kidneys store the body's energy or life power. And they are seen as the source of creativity, softness or gentleness and the overall ease or flow of life. The energy of the kidneys thus plays a key role, not just in our lives but in our liveliness—our expressiveness, our inner and outer movements—both the inner functions of our body and the outer expressions of our life.

Our sexual energy is also deeply connected to our kidneys. If the kidneys become weak, a man's health and his erections become weak and flaccid. Kidney problems can result in impotence. In order to improve your sexual power and creativity, it's vital that you care for your kidneys. When we look at the kidneys through the eyes of Western medicine and physiology, we see them primarily as filters. Automobiles also have filters—fuel filters, air filters—which stop or catch the dirt and debris before it can harm the engine. Your kidneys work in a similar way, filtering out waste products that the body disposes of through urination.

To improve your sexual health, look to your kidneys. For overall health, you should also pay heed to the liver, which is like the body's commanding general. Given the focus of this book, we'll be concentrating on the kidneys. In

Chinese medicine, it's said that the "Kidneys rule water." This includes all fluids, moisture, perspiration, blood, semen, etc.

We are most concerned about the last of these, the semen. Sperm counts and the amount of semen are directly related to your overall health—physical, emotional and mental. Simply drinking eight glasses of "alkalized ionized water" every day will help invigorate your kidneys—and will encourage them to excrete more toxins from your body, which will benefit your overall health.

Visit http://energywaterforhealth.com/ and learn about the healthful power of water.

Drinking good water will increase your sperm count, strengthen your erection and increase the electrical power that flows between the kidneys and testicles (as well as throughout your entire body).

LOCATION OF THE KIDNEYS

Your kidneys are located in your lower abdomen against your back, to the left and right side of your spine. The top of each kidney reaches to just below your lowest ribs.

A. WARMING THE HANDS METHOD

Before you touch the back area to rub your kidneys, it is very important that your hands be warm or hot. If your hands are cool or cold, you can short out or discharge the energy that's stored in your kidneys.

1. Place your hands palm-to-palm with your fingers interlaced so you can massage the palm side of the fingers as well as the palm.

2. Rub your hands together vigorously until your palms and fingers feel warm.

4. Rub your hands for about a minute.

5. Rest and feel the warmth. After you feel the warmth in your palms and fingers, it's important to relax, stop rubbing the hands and just feel the warmth.

6. Repeat this exercise until you feel warmth in your hands.

You may repeat this exercise throughout the day even in a public place.

SHAKING THE HANDS METHOD

Shaking your hands helps relax the hands, arms and shoulders. Shaking the hands also helps increase blood flow and energy. When you shake your hands, think of shaking out a wet towel, with the snapping action taking place in your fingers, palms and wrists.

1. In a sitting or standing position, bend your elbows so you raise your hands between the navel and shoulder level of your torso.

2. Start to shake your hands. This movement should be done very fast like a bird or a bee fluttering its wings.

4. Continue shaking your hands for about 1 minute.

5. Rest and feel the warmth. When you stop shaking your hands, you may feel tingling and warmth. When you feel this warmth in your palms and fingers, it's important to relax into this sensation.

6. Repeat this exercise until you feel warmth or tingling in your hands.

You may repeat this exercise throughout the day, even in a public place.

B. KIDNEY MASSAGE

Now that your palms are warm, you can use this warm current of energy in your hands to invigorate your kidneys.

1. Place your warm palms over each kidney.

2. Feel the heat flowing from the palms into the kidneys.

3. Start to rub your kidneys by moving your hands up and down over them.

4. Rub your kidneys about 18 or 36 times and rest, holding the kidneys for at least one minute or more.

5. Repeat this exercise three times.

C. KIDNEY TAPPING

When you gently tap your kidneys, you help break up and release any toxic build-up or tightness from stress or chemicals that may have accumulated in your kidneys. Doing so also releases stored emotions, such as fear, that can often be trapped in the kidneys. To tap the kidneys:

1. Make a soft fist.

2. Tap the kidneys 18 or 36 times with the back of your soft fists.

3. Rest with palms on over the kidneys, gently covering or holding the kidneys.

4. Repeat this exercise three times.

Congratulations! You have just completed the activation of your kidneys. Practice these exercises daily. Not only will they improve your sexual power, they'll have a profound, positive effect on your life overall.

FOR A MORE IN-DEPTH CONNECTION AND UNDERSTANDING, HEAR AND SEE OUR AUDIO AND VIDEO SERIES

When you join our Elite Membership site, you'll gain access to our audio and video library, which will enhance your learning experience. Plus, you'll get bonus information that will enable you to become a master in the art of lovemaking.

Go to:

http://www.BuildingYourSexualStamina.com/member

10
STEP 3—TESTICLE ACTIVATION MASSAGE

When was the last time you took the time to massage your testicles? There is power in the testicles. Your testicles produce the most important male hormone, testosterone. Testosterone enables you to feel strong, bold and powerful. Testicle massage increases the production of testosterone and the release of your sexual energy. As you learn to cultivate your testosterone, you'll increase your sexual stamina, strength and longevity.

Practicing the correct method of massaging your testicles will also increase the flow of blood into the testicular region. And it will help smooth stiff tissues (important in combating testicular cancer, cysts and benign growths). By increasing the blood flow—and in combination with the Focused-Power Breathing Method®—you will increase the flow of energy into the testicles, which will strengthen your erection and help elongate the penis.

It's very important to start with warm hands. By warming your hands before massaging your testicles, you will help stimulate more blood flow into your testicles (and throughout your body). Cold hands can shock and block your energy flow. They can make you recoil and pull away from the touch. And they indicate circulation problems. Think about it this way, would you rather have someone with nice warm hands—or with icy cold hands—massaging your back?

It's very important to have and keep warm hands. Warm hands also go a long way when touching and relaxing your partner. If you tend to have cold hands and feet, certain herbs, foods and dietary changes can help improve circulation throughout the body. (See Resource Guide, page 178.)

When massaging your testicles, the warmth from your hands will help relax and release stress from your testicles. Yes, you even have stress in your testicles. You can massage this stress away or have it massaged out in order to free 100% of your sexual power.

PRE-TESTICLE MASSAGE PREPARATION

A. Warm the Hands (see Chapter 9, STEP 2)

B. Kidney Massage (see Chapter 9, STEP 2)

C. Tap the Kidneys (see Chapter 9, STEP 2)

FINGERTIP TESTICLE MASSAGE

With warm hands, cup your testicles and hold them for about 1 minute.

1. Hold one testicle with your thumb and fingers of each hand (left testicle with left fingers—right testicle with right fingers).

2. Next, gently start massaging the testicles, using your thumb and fingers and gradually adding gentle pressure.

3. Start off softly and slowly, feeling for roundness, oval shape, hardness and any bumps or tender or sore spots. You may not be able to see these, but you can feel them with your fingers and visualize them in your mind. Don't be upset or worry about what you might find. Tenderness, pain or odd shapes will greatly improve (along with your overall health) as you massage your testicles over time.

4. Continue massaging for 3 to 5 minutes.

5. Rest and continue to cup and hold the testicles very gently.

6. Feel the warmth flowing from your hands into each testicle.

7. Repeat the Fingertip Testicle Massage 3 times.

Additional note on holding the testicles:
Hold one testicle with the fingers and palm of each hand. Now feel the warmth from your fingers and palms flowing into the testicles. Hold the testicles for about 3 minutes or more.

CONCLUSION

Repeat this sequence 3 to 5 times. You should practice this once a day for the rest of your life. If you want to become a dramatically better lover in a short period of time, then practice it twice a day. If you have health challenges, pre-ejaculation or impotence, practice these exercises three or more times daily.

FOR A MORE IN-DEPTH CONNECTION AND UNDERSTANDING, HEAR AND SEE OUR AUDIO AND VIDEO SERIES

When you join our Elite Membership site, you'll gain access to our audio and video library, which will enhance your learning experience. Plus, you'll get bonus information that will enable you to become a master in the art of lovemaking.

Go to:

http://www.BuildingYourSexualStamina.com/member

11
STEP 4—TESTICLE BREATHING METHOD

Yes, you are reading correctly—testicle breathing! And yes, it's for real. It's an art that every man should know, and any man **must** know if he wants to take command of his sexual energy.

Now you may be wondering, "Why is it that I've never heard of testicle breathing before?" Simply put, it has been a secret, closely guarded from ancient times, in certain Taoist monasteries in China. That secret has only recently been passed on to the larger world. Even in the Taoist monasteries, this knowledge was not shared with students until they had become proficient in all the preliminary stages of spiritual growth, martial arts training and so forth.

After I was trained and certified to teach these various methods, I found that the ability to harness this energy was essential not only for one's spiritual growth and for the inner martial artist to be, but equally so for the man who wanted consistent victories in the bedroom.

In the bedroom, most men fail miserably ... even if they succeed in bringing their partner to orgasm ... even if they feel moments of satisfaction at ejaculation. Still, they experience what the ancients called the "little death." After ejaculation, an overwhelming majority of men become not just sleepy but despondent—and emotionally such men become even less available to their partners.

Men are usually so weakened after ejaculating that they can barely keep their eyes open, let alone manage another erection. Being able to achieve another erection can take anywhere hours or longer—even days for some men.

THE CHOICE TO EJACULATE OR NOT TO EJACULATE

Why should a man refrain from ejaculating after the woman has climaxed? The reason is simple: There is still another level of sensual ecstasy waiting for the two of you to discover. When a man learns to have an orgasm, keep his erection and not ejaculate, his vibratory energy is multiplied.

This increases the power of his orgasm and allows him to go deeper into his sexual experience and energy. The more you are able to continue experiencing this type of inner orgasm, the higher your energy rises. And as a result, your partner is also able to experience deeper, more intense lovemaking, taking her places that, consciously or unconsciously, she has wanted to go—but never knew a man who could take her there. When your energy starts to rise, hers will rise as well, opening her heart.

Emotionally, she will pull at you from deep within. Her body will intertwine with yours, undulating uncontrollably, and her mind and body will seem like they're on fire. At this point, she'll ache for something deeper to fulfill her. You might think that she wants you—perhaps, but she's actually on the verge of opening a new doorway that will enable her to release vast amounts of negativity, bringing her closer to the essence of her soul. Together you become the vehicle for this profound, mutual experience. So hold on. Don't release. Don't ejaculate now—not when she's so close.

When she finally explodes and cries out from somewhere deep within, it will be a release so real that she may laugh with ecstasy or weep uncontrollably. But when it happens, she won't be able to hold back. She will have entered a zone of abandoning control. She'll have been released from any inhibitions, any emotional rigidity or reluctance that may once have limited her mind and body. She will have tasted the freedom of awakening to her inner source of power, and she'll always remember and thank you for taking her across that self-imposed boundary into a deeper orgasmic experience.

PRE-TESTICLE BREATHING

This is where the first stage of your internal training begins. For it is within testicle breathing that you learn to sense and feel your breath flowing in and out of your testicles. And this is a key to cultivating your sexual energy.

If you've been following the outline of this book you should be able to:

1. Feel energy with your hands.

2. Massage, tap and make your kidneys warm.

3. Massage your testicles and feel the energy.

THE ART OF TESTICLE BREATHING

To breathe into your testicles is simple. You have been breathing into every part of your body your entire life. So relax. What makes this exercise so different? You're simply going to become conscious of your breath and its movement in and out of your testicles. You'll start to feel cold or very warm energy in your testicles, as well as a tingling sensation as you draw your breath in and out of your testicles.

To begin, sit comfortably on a chair with the lower half of your body exposed. You can wear a top in order to keep the upper half of your body warm. It's better to be in an enclosed room that's very comfortable ... neither too cool nor too hot.

Please Note:
Practice these methods every day. It may take time before you feel the subtle energies in your body; however, you will prevail.

TESTICLE BREATHING METHOD

1. Sit comfortably on a chair with your scrotum hanging freely over the chair.

2. Place your tongue to the roof of your mouth tongue behind your upper teeth.

3. Rest with your palms on your thighs.

4. Hold your head even, as if you are hanging by a string from the center point or top of your head.

5. Gently tuck your chin, which raises the back of your head.

6. Smile with your lips and feel your entire body smile. (This is very important.)

7. Become aware of a sensation within your testicles.

8. Spiral this sensation in small circles with your mind on and into your testicles for 2 minutes.

   SUMMARY:

   A. Visualize and feel very small circles or spirals of energy moving across or through each testicle.

B Take your time. It may take several sessions before you can feel and make a real connection with your testicles.

9. Inhale slowly through your nose into your testicles, as you gently pull or lift your testicles up by squeezing your perineum or anal sphincter muscles.

SUMMARY:

A. Squeeze and pull your anus up into your body, towards the top of your head.
B. This should take about 4 to 7 seconds. (As you do so, your testicles will move or lift up closer towards your body.)
C. This movement may be very slight in the beginning. However, it will become more noticeable as you grow stronger over time.

See Illustration on Next Page

TESTICLE BREATHING

Spine

Coccyx

INHALE, DRAW ENERGY INTO THE TESTICLES

10. Hold your breath and hold your testicles up, for 3 to 5 seconds.

11. Exhale slowly through the nose and slowly release and lower the testicles back down. (This should take about 4 to 7 seconds.)

12. Feel the cool energy in the scrotum.

13. Repeat this exercise (points 9–12), doing so 9 times.

Rest for 30 seconds, and feel the cool or magnetic energy in the scrotal area.

EXHALE INTO THE PERINUM

1. Inhale slowly through your nose into your testicles as you gently pull or lift your testicles upward by gently squeezing your perineum or anal sphincter muscles. (See "Testicle Breathing," above.)

SUMMARY:

A. Squeeze and pull your anus upward into your body, toward the top of your head.

B. This should take about 4 to 7 seconds. (Your testicles will move or lift closer to your body.)

C. This movement may be very slight in the beginning. However, it will become more noticeable as you grow stronger over time.

2. Hold your breath, and continue drawing your testicles up. (Hold for 3 to 5 seconds.)

3. Exhale slowly through the nose, and slowly release and lower your testicles. (This should take about 4 to 7 seconds.)

4. Feel the cool energy flowing from the testicles into the perineum as you exhale. (See "Exhaling Energy into the Perineum," below.)

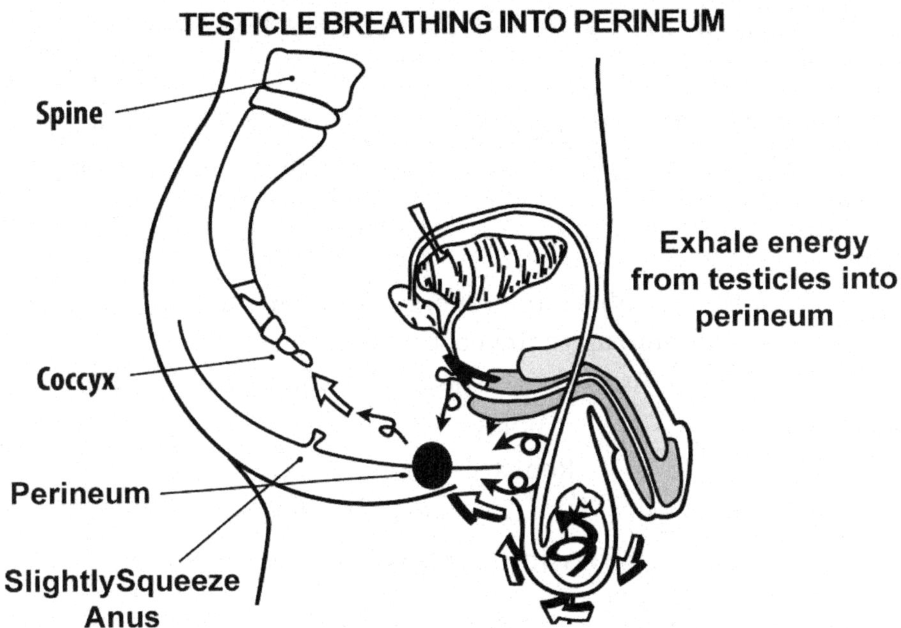

5. Repeat this exercise (points 1–4) 9 times.

6. Rest and feel the cool or magnetic energy in the scrotal and perineum area. (Rest for 30 seconds.)

The non-aroused and aroused sexual energy will flow from the navel center, down into the testicles, up the back of the spine and into the head

BREATHING TESTICLE ENERGY UP THE SPINE

Refer back to the illustration, "Moving the Cool Sexual Energy up the Spine," as you address the various levels that follow.

1. Gently inhale this energy from the testicles and perineum up to the coccyx (Level 1).
    - A. Exhale into the coccyx and sacrum point.
    - B. Repeat 3 times.

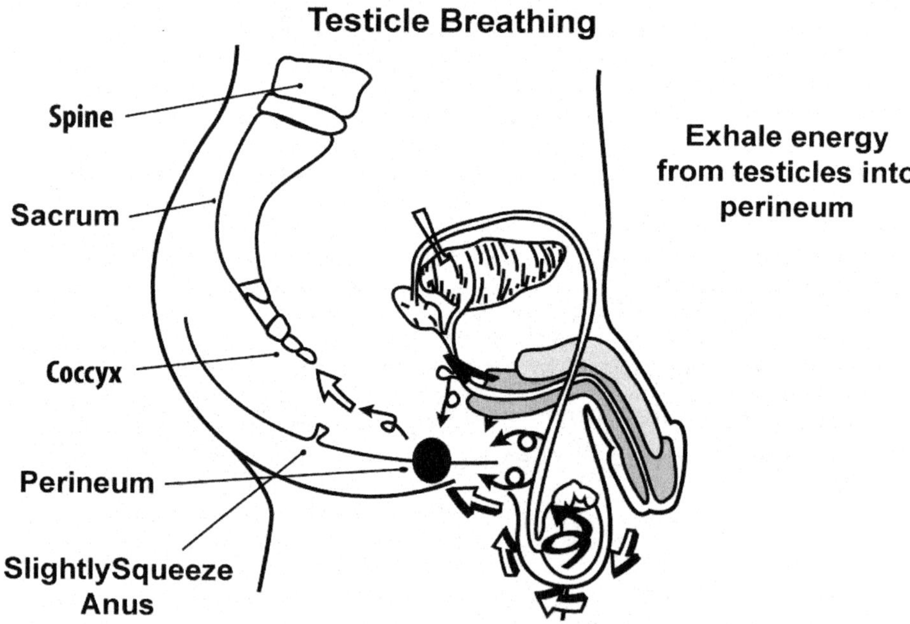

2. Gently inhale this energy from the testicles up to the sacrum (Level 2).
    A. Exhale into the sacrum.
    B. Repeat 3 times.

3. Gently inhale this energy from the testicles up to the kidney point (Level 3).
    A. Exhale into the kidney point.
    B. Repeat 3 times.

4. Gently inhale this energy from the testicles up to T11 (Level 4).
    A. Exhale into T11.
    B. Repeat 3 times.

5. Gently inhale this energy from the testicles up to the back of the heart (Level 5).
    A. Exhale into the back of the heart.
    B. Repeat 3 times

6. Gently inhale this energy from the testicles up to C7 (Level 6).
    A. Exhale into C7.
    B. Repeat 3 times.

7. Gently inhale this energy from the testicles up to jade pillow or base of the skull (Level 7).
    A. Exhale into the base of skull.
    B. Repeat 3 times.

8. Gently inhale this energy from the testicles up to the crown (Level 8).
    A. Exhale into the crown.
    B. Repeat 3 times.

9. Gently inhale this energy from the testicles up the spine to the top of your head.
    A. Exhale into the crown.
    B. Repeat 3 times.

10. Rest with this energy in your head.
    A. Rest for 3 to 5 minutes.
    B. As you gently inhale, expand your stomach area, and feel your breath/air enter into your testicles. (Inhale this way for about 5 to 7 seconds.)
    C. As you exhale, feel your testicles filling up with more energy. Feel and become confident that you are breathing into your testicles. In time, it will become more real and undeniably true that your testicles do breath.

Repeat this routine once or twice a day for the rest of your life.

Here are a few of the benefits of testicle breathing: It improves your erection, giving you firmness and hardness; it slows the aging process; it increases and balances your inner energy.

FOR A MORE IN-DEPTH CONNECTION AND UNDERSTANDING, HEAR AND SEE OUR AUDIO AND VIDEO SERIES

When you join our Elite Membership site, you'll gain access to our audio and video library, which will enhance your learning experience. Plus, you'll get bonus information that will enable you to become a master in the art of lovemaking.

Go to:

http://www.BuildingYourSexualStamina.com/member

12
STEP 5—SCROTUM COMPRESSION BREATHING METHOD

The Scrotum Compression Breathing Method enables you to condense your sexual energy into the scrotum area. This method will increase your sexual energy and prolong your ability to handle sexual excitement. Compression Breathing reduces and, over time, eliminates premature ejaculation and nocturnal emissions.

THREE-CENTER ACTIVATION

Before we begin the Scrotum Compression exercises, we will begin by activating the three centers. The three centers are located at the throat, solar plexus and testicles/scrotum. It is best to practice this exercise sitting or standing until you have gained a degree of proficiency.

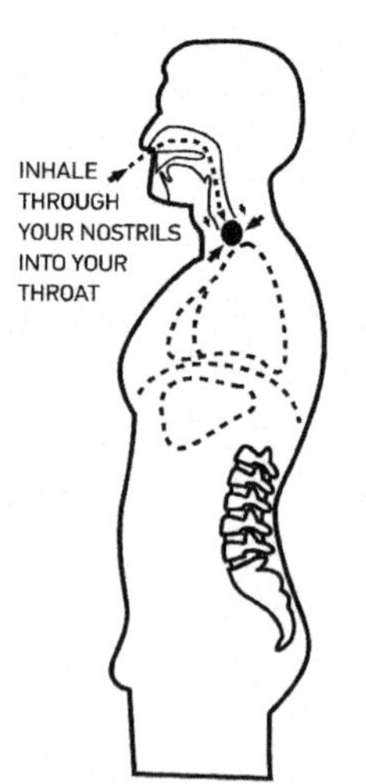

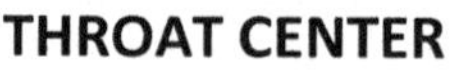
THROAT CENTER

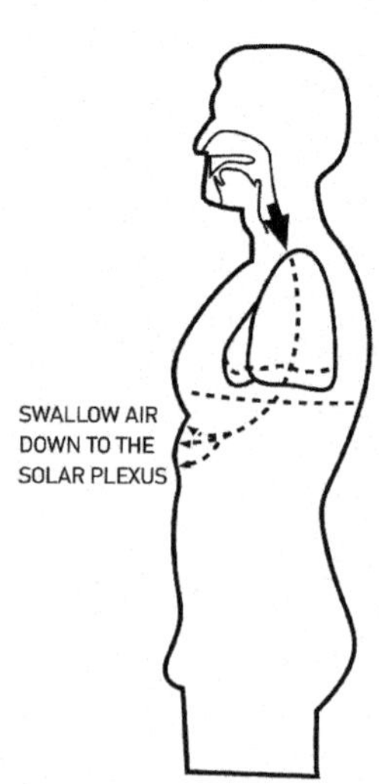

SOLAR PLEXUS CENTER

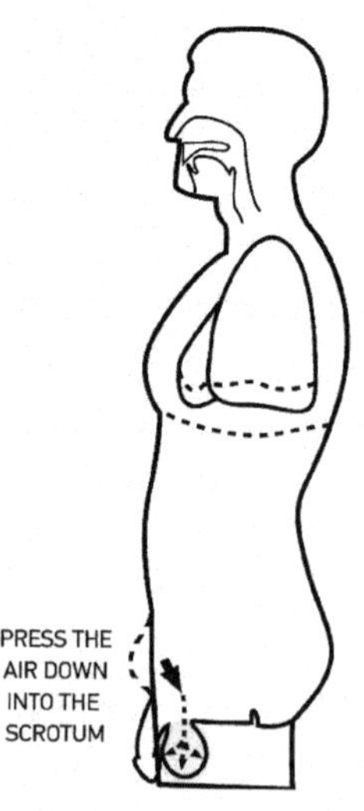

TESTICLE CENTER

THREE-CENTER ACTIVATION

1. Inhale a large amount of air into your throat.

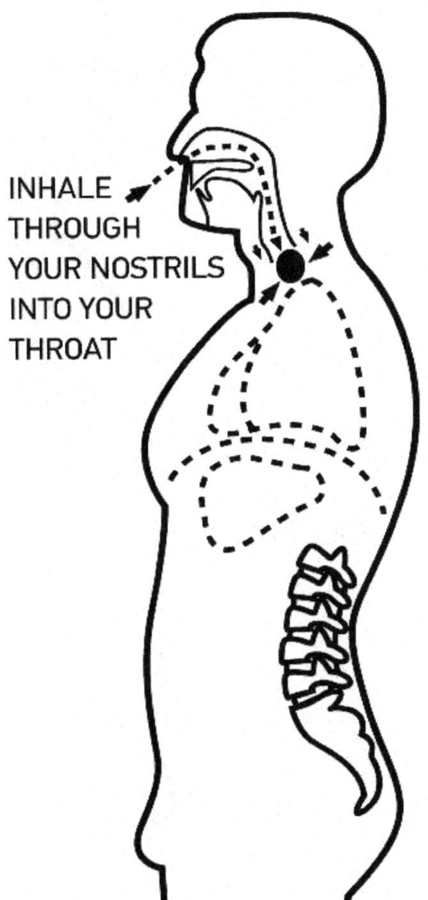

2. Hold your breath.

3. Swallow and drive or roll this air from the throat down into the solar plexus and hold it there.

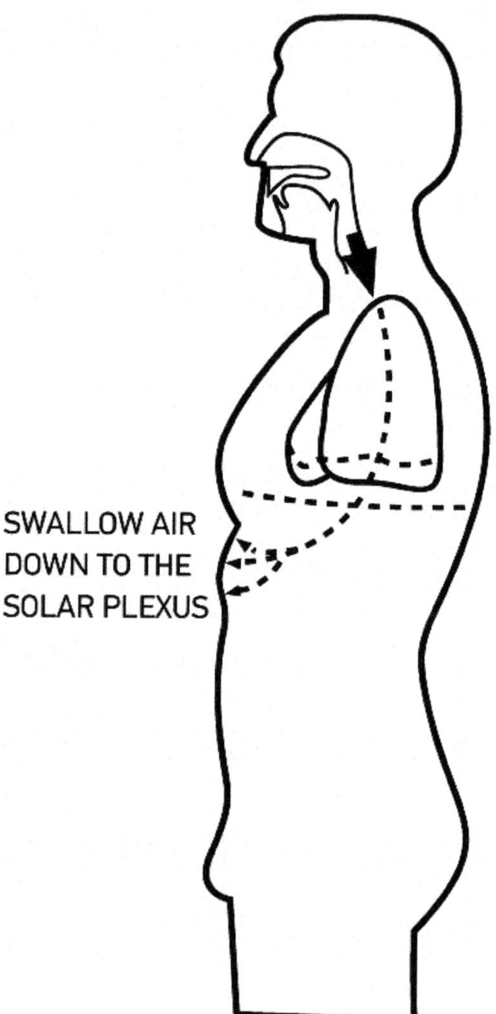

4. Continue to hold your breath.

5. Swallow again and drive or roll this air from the solar plexus down to the testicles.

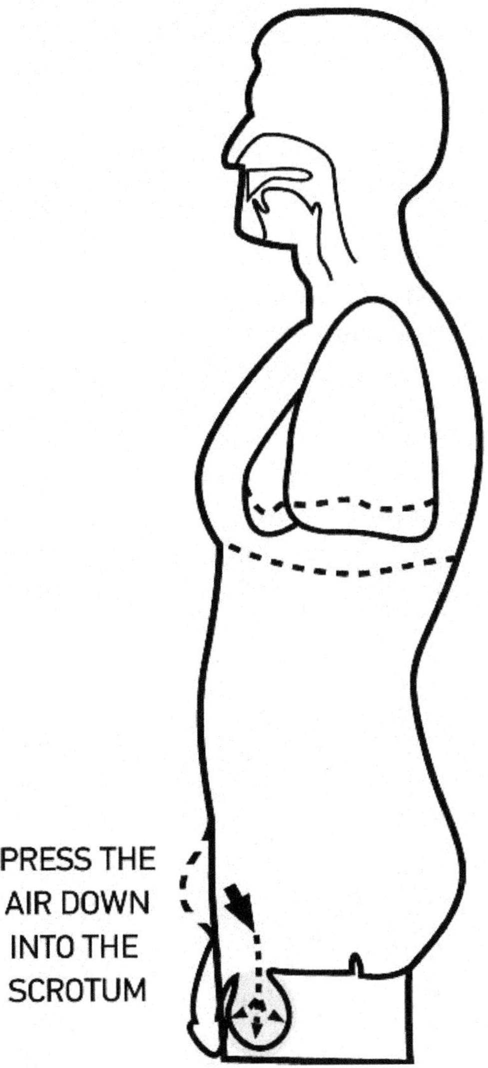

A. Continue to hold your breath.

B. Count to 6.

6. Slowly exhale and feel the air leaving the lower abdominal area, solar plexus, upper chest and nose.

Relax. As you swallow and push the air through your three centers (throat, solar plexus and scrotum), allow your diaphragm to accomplish this by contracting and releasing your abdominal muscles in a wavelike motion downward into the testicles.

When the air reaches the testicles you may feel a movement of heat flowing to various points and places in your body. You may notice that your testicles expand as you compress the air down.

As you become more adept at driving air into your testicles, you may feel the energy flowing up your spine. Every time you perform the Scrotal Compression exercise, you're shooting tremendous energy into the testicles. Doing so halts energy loss and premature ejaculations.

THE COMPLETE SCROTAL COMPRESSION BREATHING METHOD—WARNING:

You should not overexert yourself while performing these breathing exercises. You do not need to hold your breath throughout the exercises, as outlined. You should feel free to exhale or inhale at any given point. DO NOT PASS OUT. If you take your time, over time you'll be able to perform the Complete Scrotal Compression Exercise Breathing Method with ease and power. I cannot emphasize this enough: Do not strain yourself. If you feel dizzy or faint, stop and rest. Dizziness is an indication that you are trying too hard or taking on more than you are capable of at this time. Be gentle and patient. Remember that I also offer online audio and video tapes to assist you at:

http://www.BuildingYourSexualStamina.com/member

THE COMPLETE SCROTAL COMPRESSION BREATHING METHOD INSTRUCTIONS

1. Sit on the edge of a chair. You can wear loose-fitting clothes or pants or nothing at all from the waist down so your testicles can hang freely.

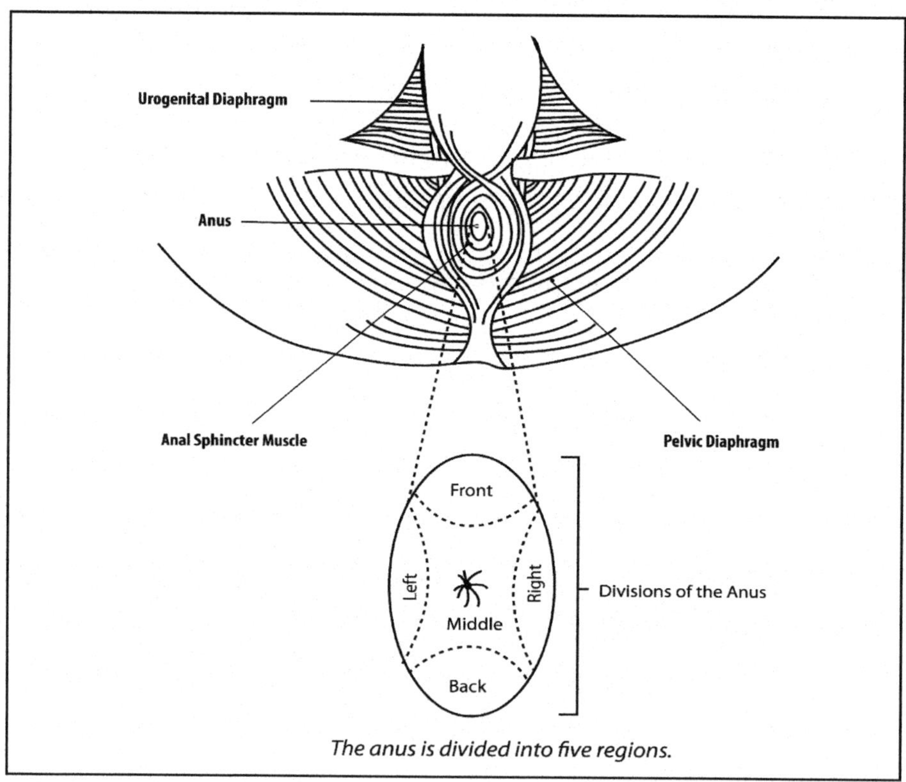

The anus is divided into five regions.

2. Place your feet flat on the floor and about a shoulder-width apart.
3. Tighten and close the anus/anal sphincter and the perineum muscle during the entire sequence.
4. Very quickly, inhale a large amount of air into the throat center. Breathe through your nose only.

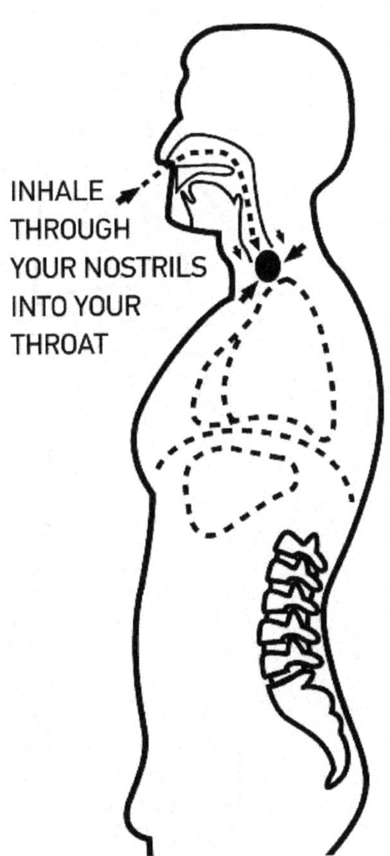

5. Hold the breath in your throat area.

6. While still holding your breath, swallow some saliva, pushing it down and making a gulping sound.

7. Now drive or roll the inhaled air from your throat down into your solar plexus. Feel the air like a ball.

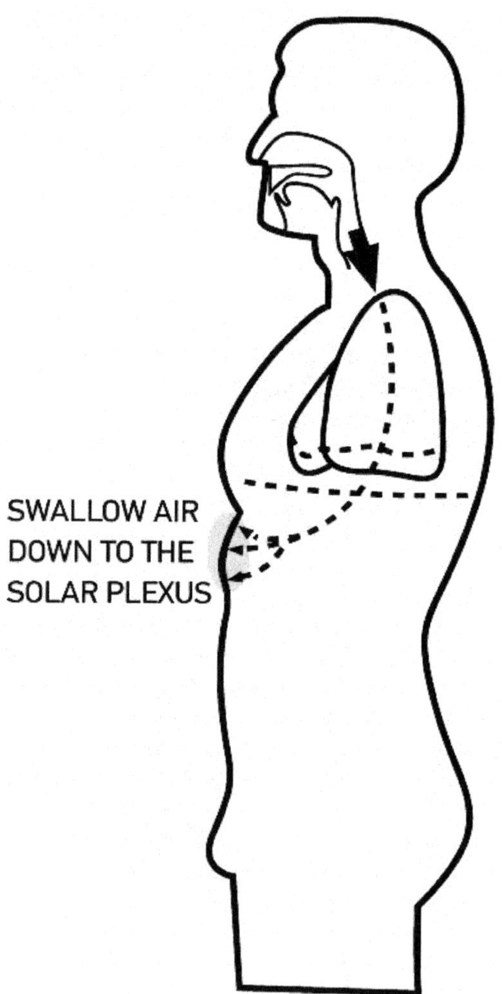

8. Hold the breath in the solar plexus area.

9. Roll the ball from the solar plexus down to the navel.

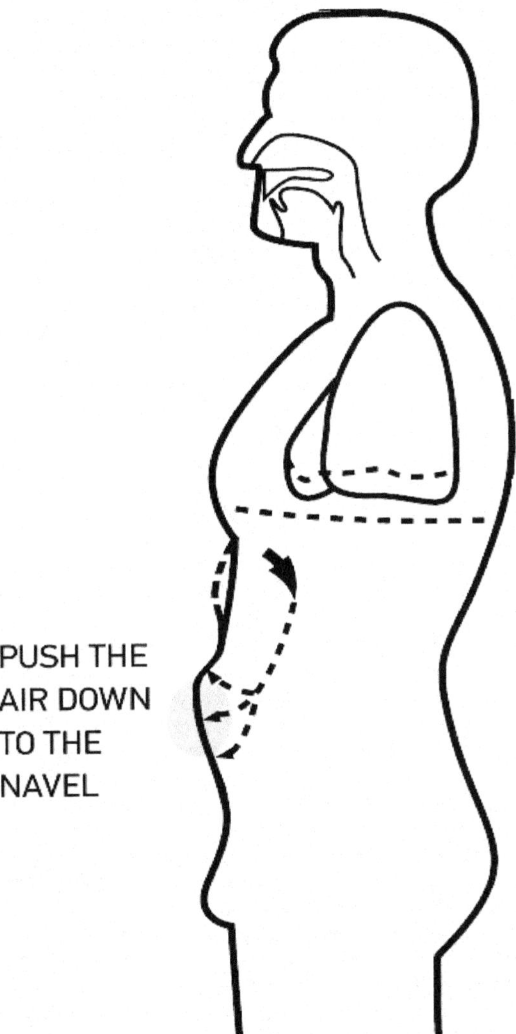

10. Hold the breath in the navel area.

11. Roll the ball of air from the navel area into the pelvic area, prostate and bladder.

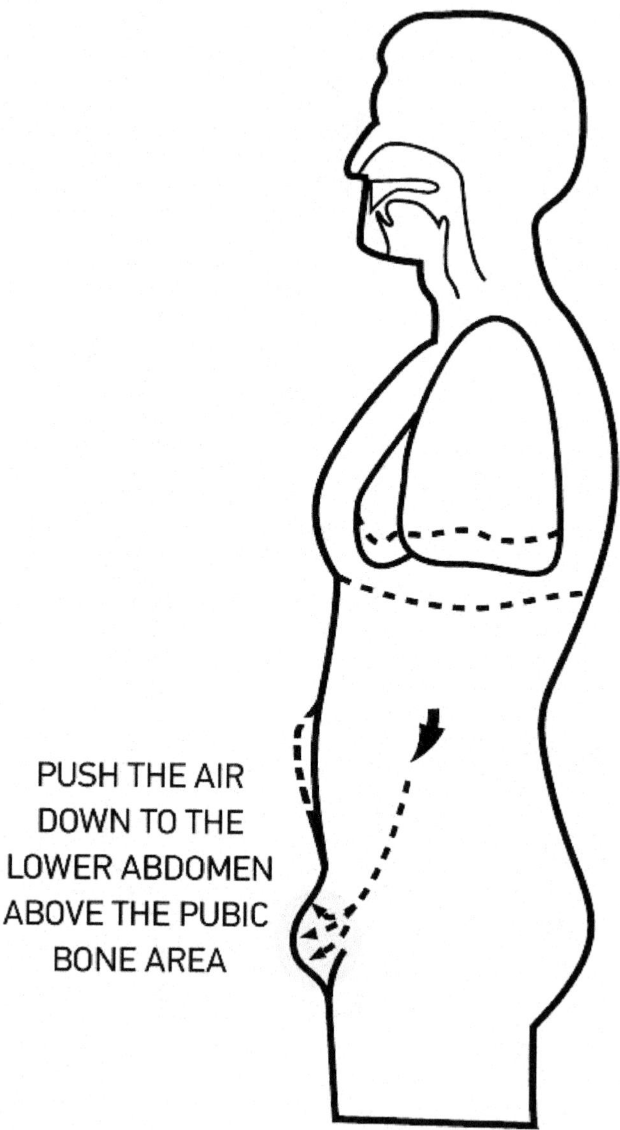

12. Hold the breath in the pelvic area.

13. Roll the ball of air from the pelvic area into the scrotum and testicles.

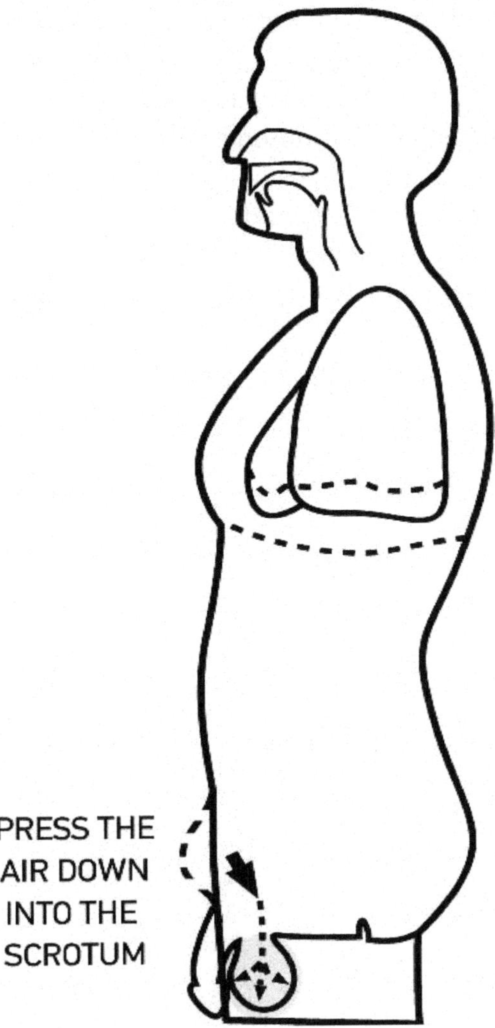

14. Forcibly push, hold and compress the air into the scrotum for as long as you can.

15. Try to hold the compressed air there, initially for about 10 to 30 seconds. Slowly build your time up to a full minute.

16. Swallow any saliva that may have accumulated.

17. Slowly exhale and relax. Release the anus (anal sphincter) and perineum muscle.

18. Rest for 30 to 60 seconds.

19. Repeat the exercise (points 3–18), doing so 3, 6, 9, 18 or 36 times.

COOL YOUR BODY AND REGAIN YOUR COMPOSURE WITH RAPID-FIRE BREATHING

Rapid-Fire Breathing is designed to quickly activate the qi (energy) in the lower abdominal area. Rapid-Fire Breathing can also cool and balance the energy throughout your body. Breathing with Rapid-Fire Breathing draws energy into the testicle area for an erection. The stronger the breath that flows into the lower abdomen area, the stronger the blood flow. And the stronger the blood flow, the more qi (energy) will me gathered for your erection.

Breathing with Rapid-Fire Breathing can also help cool and disperse the intense sexual energy before ejaculation. Rapid-Fire Breathing speeds up the number of breaths by at least 3 to 1 so, within a 5 second span, you can have 15 to 20 quick breaths, counting both inhalations and exhalations.

THE RAPID-FIRE BREATHING METHOD

1. Inhale and exhale 45 to 60 times over 15 seconds. Be aware of your abdomen moving in and out as your breath moves in and out. Remember: When you inhale, your abdomen moves out or expands; when you exhale, it flattens or compresses.

2. Rest for 15 seconds.

3. Repeat 4 times.

SUMMARY OF THE SCROTAL COMPRESSION BREATHING METHOD

1. Stand or sit and keep your alignment straight and your tongue to the roof of your mouth.

2. Breathe in through your nose, drawing your breath into the throat.

3. Swallow and push the air down into the solar plexus.

4. Continue pressing the ball of air down into the navel area.

5. Press the ball of air from the navel area down into the pelvic area.

6. Next, press the ball of air into the scrotum, until you can hold your breath no longer.

7. At the end of holding your breath, swallow your saliva, making a gulping sound as you were forcibly pushing your salvia down.

8. Exhale slowly through your nose.

9. Rest by performing Rapid-Fire Breathing.

10. Stand, stretch and rotate your waist in a circle 3, 6 or 9 times.

11. Repeat 1–10.

Start with 5 Scrotal Compression Breathing Exercises and slowly increase to 36.

FOR A MORE IN-DEPTH CONNECTION AND UNDERSTANDING, HEAR AND SEE OUR AUDIO AND VIDEO SERIES

When you join our Elite Membership site, you'll gain access to our audio and video library, which will enhance your learning experience. Plus, you'll get bonus information that will enable you to become a master in the art of lovemaking.

Go to:

http://www.BuildingYourSexualStamina.com/member

Use our members-only Scrotum Compression Breathing CDs, videos, and audios to increase your sexual stamina and strength. Watch, listen and learn—step by step—how to master these vital exercises.—Walter

13
STEP 6—SELF-CULTIVATION: ENERGETIC MASTURBATION

The ancient way to fuller understanding of the art of sexual empowerment involved spending hundreds or thousands of hours alone, learning to gain mastery over one's sexual energy. This solitary training is called self- or single-cultivation. After reaching a certain level of proficiency, the person would also spend as much time, if not more, in dual cultivation with another person.

MASTURBATION VERSUS SELF-CULTIVATION

As generally understood, masturbation is the act of stimulating oneself in a sexual way in order to experience orgasm and ejaculation. However, self-cultivation differs from masturbation. Although both involve the act of self-stimulation, self-cultivation does not have a conclusion or ejaculation as its goal. The purpose of self-cultivation as outlined in this book is to teach men to:

1. Experience prolonged sexual stimulation without going over the edge or ejaculating.
2. Have multiple orgasms without ejaculating.
3. Direct and channel their sexual energy.

Stimulation or arousal can be achieved by using your hand(s) or through the assistance of another person or by using sexual aids or devices.

SELF-CULTIVATION OR ENERGETIC MASTURBATION

In other words, self-cultivation or energetic masturbation involves sexual stimulation. The goal is not simply to stimulate yourself sexually but to activate and feel your arousal energy—and to cultivate the relationship between your mind, body functions and sexual energy. Unlike simple masturbation, the goal isn't "release"—rather it's gaining mastery or command over the flow of sexual energy through your body.

The methods you are about to learn will enable you to take command of the subtle movement of your sexual energy. By means of specific muscle contractions and the focused power of your mind, you'll be able to direct that energy through your body. In particular, you'll learn to move sexual energy away from your penis—gathering, dispersing and re-gathering that energy as you choose. Finally, it's important to realize that moving your sexual energy in this fashion has added benefits, besides letting you extend your lovemaking: It will also strengthen and re-energize your body overall.

Men who learn to move their sexual energy away from their penis and into their spine learn that doing so energizes the nervous system, which feeds the brain, organs, glands, skeletal, muscular, respiratory, senses, vascular, immune, lymph and digestive systems.

SELF-STIMULATION AND SELF-CULTIVATION

The practice of self cultivation can be divided into three parts:

1. **Attention**
2. **Discipline**
3. **Consistency**

Attention

By focusing your attention on your body and carefully following the inner flow of your energy or stimulation, you will start to feel—and learn to direct—your sexual energy. However, when you focus your energy on someone else (this includes pictures or fantasies) your energy will flow into that outward person or object. Sending sexual energy into your partner is a desirable goal—indeed, one of the highest—however, to reap the full benefits, you must first learn to control and direct the energy within yourself. So, this first level of exercises in watching and commanding our sexual energy requires that you separate yourself from your partner, from images and fantasies, and focus wholly on yourself.

As you stimulate yourself in these exercises, feel your arousal energy, but be careful not to go too close to the edge. The goal is to stimulate but not **overstimulate** (and ejaculate). If you do ejaculate, this part of your training will be over. However, you can begin again after a six-hour wait.

Discipline

You'll need discipline to push past your desire to ejaculate and release the perceived pressure of your arousal. Discipline implies both restraint and skills—not only knowing what to do but also when to let go. It will take willpower and determination to resist the urge to ejaculate. But you need to accustom yourself to doing so. By understanding and controlling your intense feelings as you approach that point—using the systematic methods outlined in this book—you'll be training yourself, body, mind and emotions, how to use your supercharged sexual energy.

The key to using your sexual energy is being able to separate your arousal from ejaculation—so you enjoy the great pleasure of your arousal energy while resisting the urge to ejaculate. This discipline is the key to unleashing the power of full, unselfish sex.

Consistency

The only way to master the art of love is through proper attention, discipline and consistency. Consistency along with attention and discipline (or skill) will determine your success and or failure. For best results, spend about 15 to 30 minutes once or twice a day cultivating your sexual arousal energy.

SELF-CULTIVATION DAILY PRACTICE

When you experience the feelings you feel just before you ejaculate reaching the 80% to 95% mark, you must STOP. Don't go too far into the ejaculation feeling or mode.

Rest and breathe in using Rapid-Fire Breathing for 1 minute and then Focused-Power Breathing for 3 to 5 minutes, allowing your erection to subside.

1. Start to stimulate yourself; be aware of your penis and your arousal energy.
2. However, once you become aroused, focus your attention just on your arousal energy.
3. Cup the testicles with one hand and with the other hand make small circles around the sexual center, which is just below the navel.

Repeat this sequence 3, 5 or 9 times per practice session.

You will gain greater proficiency if you do not ejaculate for 90 days.

Be patient, and remember that your goal at this stage is learning how to avoid ejaculating even when your strong feelings seem to want you to. This isn't the endpoint: Your training will take you beyond this limited place. Learning to feel strong sensations without losing yourself is a vital step on the path to expanding your sexual powers and your enjoyment.

Note: Try not to use x-rated videos, fantasies, *Playboy* or similar magazines—learn to connect with your sexual energy without relying on such outside forms of stimulation. However if you are challenged by soft erections or you have little or no arousal sensation, you may turn to fantasies and visual aids of a lover.

FOR A MORE IN-DEPTH CONNECTION AND UNDERSTANDING, HEAR AND SEE OUR AUDIO AND VIDEO SERIES

When you join our Elite Membership site, you'll gain access to our audio and video library, which will enhance your learning experience. Plus, you'll get bonus information that will enable you to become a master in the art of lovemaking.

Go to:

http://www.BuildingYourSexualStamina.com/member

14
STEP 7—THE MILLION-DOLLAR POINT

The Million-Dollar Point is also referred to as the external locking method.

When I first learned about the Million-Dollar Point from Taoist master Mantak Chia, he stated that when you learn to apply the Million-Dollar Point properly it is invaluable. However, when you miss this point, it's not even worth a penny. When you learn to use this point correctly, it will save you from ejaculating too soon, and it will allow you to experience an inward release or reverse ejaculation. This is the most effective way of experiencing an ejaculation with very little loss of energy.

Please note: You may experience some loss of your erection, however continue to apply stimulation and the penis will become erect. Your libido or sexual drive is still available.

EJACULATION IN TWO PARTS

First, we will look at what happens when a man ejaculates. The ejection of semen occurs in two parts.

In the first phase, the **contractile (or emission) phase**, your prostate contracts and releases multiple times very quickly, emptying the semen from the prostate into the urethra.

Then, in the second, or **expulsion,** phase, your semen is pushed down the urethra and out of your penis.

When a man learns to become multi-orgasmic, he is able to have non-ejaculatory orgasms. He still has the prostate contractions or flutters. However, no external ejaculation takes place. He is able to keep his vital energy, allowing him to continue having sex while his penis maintains 60% to 70% or more of its erection and hardness.

THREE-FINGER EXTERNAL LOCKING

When you learn to press the Million-Dollar Point, you can stop your body from emptying your semen into the urethra and pushing the semen out of the penis, thus preventing an external ejaculation.

However, while holding this point and continuing to have sex, you can move into and experience a very powerful inner ejaculation. This process involves an ejaculation—but it will be a reverse ejaculation. You enter into a reverse ejaculation by holding the Million-Dollar Point. When successful at holding this point no fluids pass into or out of the penis or into the urethra. This holding of the Million-Dollar Point conserves or keeps 60% to 70% or more of your energy intact inside your body, to be reabsorbed back into the body, allowing you to maintain your vitality and ability to continue to have sex.

Pressing on the Million-Dollar Point or the perineum (the point between your anus and testicles) works because of the all-important prostate gland. When the prostate gland becomes sufficiently stimulated, either by direct or indirect means, it pulsates or flutters, and this response is at the core of a man's ejaculation.

THE SEXUAL MUSCLE GROUP

If the glands, muscles and tendons of the sexual muscle group are weak and stiff, they will be unable to hold back the tremendous forces that produce an ejaculation.

The exercise that follows will take time to learn, but once you've mastered this technique, you'll immediately see its value.

At the base of this exercise is a sensation. The feeling or quality of this sensation is somewhat like that of trying to hold back urination. To start, we will only work with the breath, prostate gland, muscles, tendons and the aroused sexual energy.

CONTRACTING THE SEXUAL MUSCLE GROUP

Let's try first to learn to contract the sexual muscle group at will. This exercise is simple, and you've probably done it a million times, particularly if you've ever felt the need to urinate but had to hold back, physically tightening the muscles around your penis to stop yourself.

Building your sexual muscle group is based on much the same technique, except without the need to urinate. To start, I want you to contract this muscle group by squeezing the anus and perineum and by closing the penis down, as if you were stopping the flow of urine. Notice what happens when you contract, the head of your penis closes down. You're using what's called a ring muscle to tighten the opening. You're also pulling up on your anus, closing another set of ring muscles as well as pulling up on the perineum. All of these ring muscles are being pulled up and tightened.

At the same time, two other, internal sets of ring muscles close—those of the bladder (which holds the urine) and the prostate (which holds the sperm after they leave the testicles).

Try squeezing, holding and releasing the perineum ring muscle. Allow yourself time and patience to experience the sensation of each of various ring muscles closing and opening.

Squeeze and release 30 times, 3 times a day for 90 days. **Note:** You can practice this exercise throughout the day.

CAUTION

To avoid hemorrhoids or other potential injuries, do not use excessive force—pushing, pulling, pressing or straining—while you perform the above exercises.

USE OF THE MILLION-DOLLAR POINT

1. Become aroused up to 70%, but don't go over the edge and ejaculate.

MILLION-DOLLAR POINT CHART

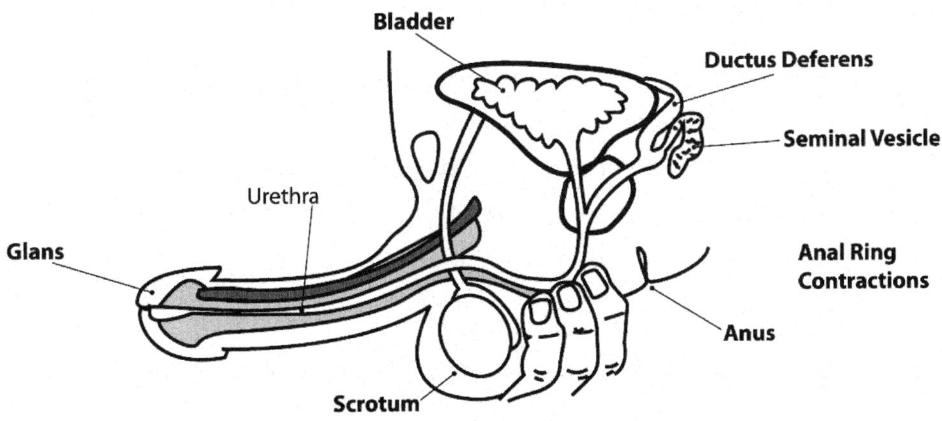

2. **Apply the three-finger method:** Bring your index, middle and ring fingers together and press them at the perineum very firmly. Using your fingers, press with a gentle force up and against the floor of your torso, that is, against your perineum.

3. Hold this point until your erection subsides and the urge to ejaculate dissipates.

4. Repeat from the beginning, progressively increasing your arousal energy—for example, allowing your arousal to reach 75% for your second try, 80% for your third, 85% for your fourth and 90% for your fifth. Each time you increase your sexual arousal energy, the stronger the urge to ejaculate will become and the more strength you will need to hold your energy within.

You can practice this method either alone or with your partner. However you may want to explain to her what you are up to as you reach down or around and start to press this point as she is riding you. (With some guidance, she can also press the point for you.)

Have fun!

CAUTION: This method is not effective for birth control. Seminal fluids may leak out.

FOR A MORE IN-DEPTH CONNECTION AND UNDERSTANDING, HEAR AND SEE OUR AUDIO AND VIDEO SERIES

When you join our Elite Membership site, you'll gain access to our audio and video library, which will enhance your learning experience. Plus, you'll get bonus information that will enable you to become a master in the art of lovemaking.

Go to:

http://www.BuildingYourSexualStamina.com/member

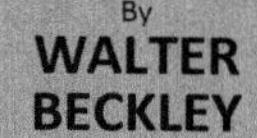

15
STEP 8—PC MUSCLE CONTRACTIONS

The pubococcygeus muscle or PC muscle is a hammock-like muscle found in both sexes that stretches from the pubic bone to the coccyx (tail bone) forming the floor of the pelvic cavity and supporting the pelvic organs. It's part of the levator ani group of muscles.

Muscle contractions lead to deeper relaxation. Muscle contractions combined with qi energy will activate more energy flow deep within the muscles, bones, tendons and blood. These muscle contractions will enhance, balance and strengthen your skeletal muscular systems.

By controlling the various muscle groups and gently stretching the tendons, you'll be able to direct the flow of your sexual energy as it increases, stops or moves too fast.

The following exercise will help you move your sexual arousal energy from your genital area into your spine and brain.

PC MUSCLE CONTRATION EXERCISE

To begin:

1. Sit in a chair or stand.

2. Lean back and relax.

3. Gently close your fist.

4. Rest your feet and toes gently against the floor.

5. As you **exhale**, start to contract your left and right hip muscles, curling your buttocks towards your thighs.

6. At the same time, with palms down, squeeze your fists together as you slowly turn them over, drawing a circle with your baby fingers, tracing an invisible line that ends with both fingers and palms facing towards the ceiling.

7. As you perform points 5 and 6, contract and squeeze, curling your toes under as if you are gripping the earth.

8. **Inhale** and relax.

9. Repeat this exercise 9 or 18 times.

Notes: You may become aware that your perineum and testicles lift slightly. You may also notice that the tip of your penis and your anus close while contracting. You may also feel your back area rounding and your chest and navel area becoming more concave.

REVERSE BREATHING CONTRACTION EXERCISE

1. Sit in a chair.

2. Lean back and relax.

3. Gently close your fist.

4. Rest your feet and toes gently against the floor.

5. As you **inhale** (reverse breathing), Start to contract your left and right hip muscles, curling your buttocks towards your thighs.

6. At the same time, with palms down, squeeze your fists together as you slowly turn them over, tracing a circle with your baby fingers that ends with both fingers and palms facing towards the ceiling.

7. As you perform points 5 and 6, contract and squeeze, curling your toes under as if you are gripping the earth.

8. Exhale and relax.

9. Repeat this exercise 9 or 18 times.

16
STEP 9—THE POWER LOCK AND ORGASMIC BIG DRAW

The purpose of the Power Lock is to stop or block your highly aroused sexual energy from being released from your body. As we discussed earlier, in "Surviving the Little Death," when a man ejaculates, he loses energy. However, by retaining this highly aroused sexual energy and learning how to move it to other parts of the body, he can increase his overall physical, mental and emotional vitality. (Sexual energy is the only energy in the body that can be increased and transformed into a higher-level energy and vibration.)

The goal of the Orgasmic Big Draw is to enable you to draw your aroused sexual energy from your genital area into other parts of your body. Doing so will result in an increase in the energy within your spine, brain, senses, organs, glands, bones, etc.

As you begin to draw your aroused sexual energy from your sexual organ, your erection will start to subside. Don't worry. After a bit of physical, mental or emotional stimulation, you will come back.

THE NEXT THREE CHARTS

The next three charts are very important for you to learn, understand and memorize. They show the relationship between particular energy points and their respective locations in your body. Revisit these charts often or until you can visualize them clearly from memory.

THE POWER LOCK—ORGASMIC BIG DRAW CHART

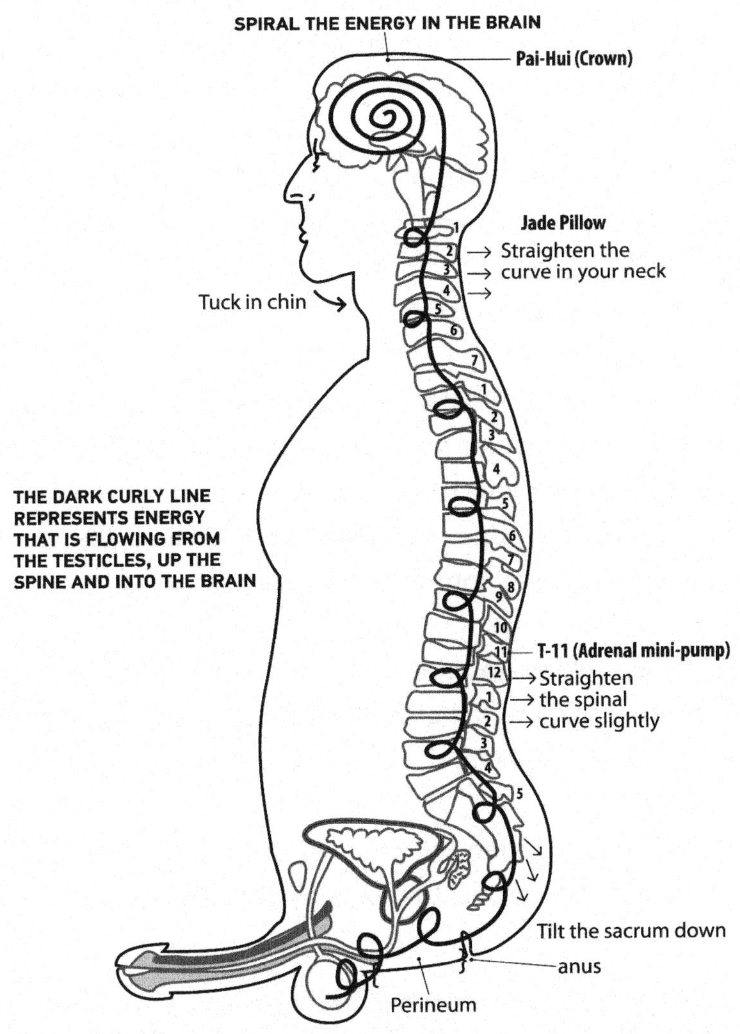

Over time, using the Power Lock together with the Orgasmic Big Draw will train your mind to draw sexual energy up into the higher-energy centers, without the use of muscular contractions.

THE POWER LOCK AND ORGASMIC BIG DRAW METHOD ACTIVATING SEXUAL ENERGY THROUGH SELF-AROUSAL

1. To begin, it's best to stand or sit. **WARNING:** Do not lay down until you gain a high level of proficiency in stopping and circulating your aroused sexual energy.

2. Become aroused up to 70%, but do not go over the edge and ejaculate. As you feel your sexual energy start to become more intense, **stop thrusting or stimulating yourself.**

The key is to stimulate yourself (your penis) to between 70% and 90% of the point of ejaculation. Do not go over the edge. Once you reach a point of no return and once you go over the edge (ejaculate), you will lose your energy and your ability to continue this exercise.

So be diligent in not getting too close to your edge. Why? Because once you fall over the edge (ejaculate), only time will allow you to be ready for further training.

3. Here's an option for the next phase: Use your mind to create the arousal energy by focusing your thoughts

on your penis and then circulating that energy around the head of your penis until you become aroused or feel some form of stimulation. This method is a more advanced technique.

ONCE YOU'RE AROUSED, WHAT THEN?

THE POWER LOCK, PART 1

Power Lock Excercise

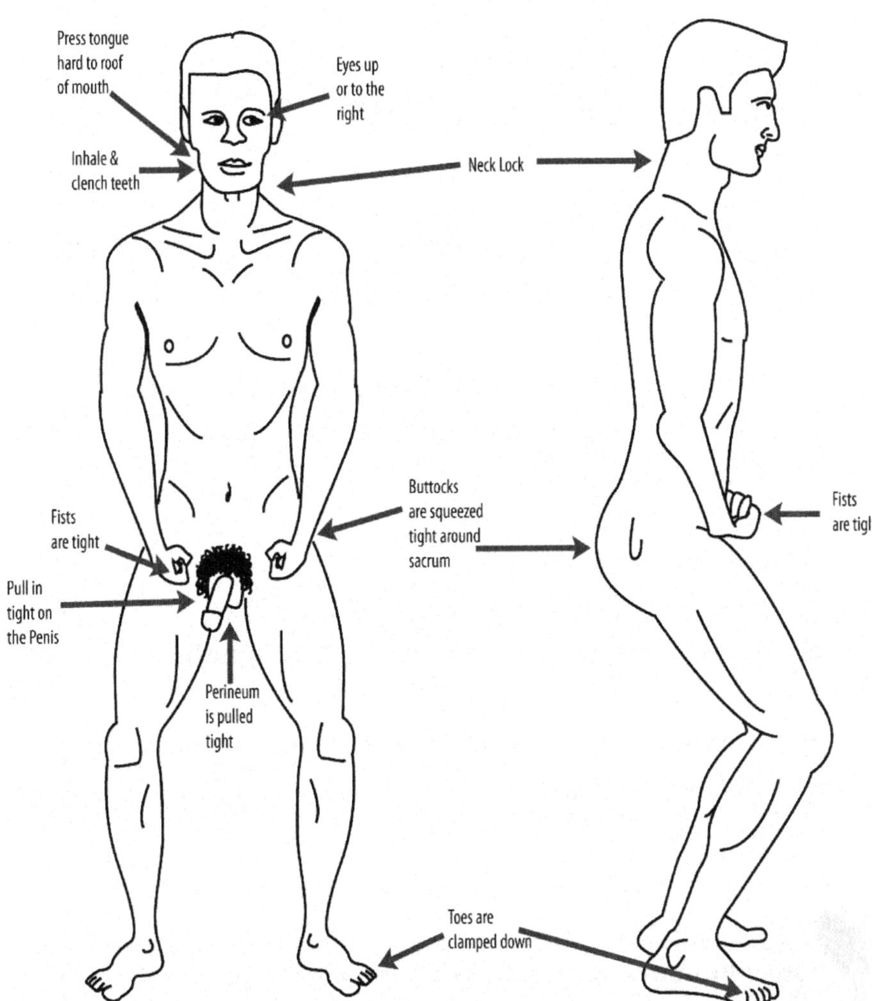

1. Inhale. (Reverse breathing—your navel should go inward toward the spine.) Inhale quickly.

    A. This should be a small breath, drawing in only about 30% of your capacity, allowing you to feel comfortable as you hold your breath through the remaining parts of the exercise.

    B. Be very gentle as you inhale and hold the air in.

    C. If you feel the need to breathe, exhale a little and take in more air. But don't release all the air.

2. Claw the earth with your feet.

3. Clench your feet.

4. Tighten your buttock muscles into your thigh muscles.

5. Draw your anus up toward the top of your head.

6. Tuck in your chin.

7. Clench your teeth.

8. Press your tongue to the roof of your mouth.

9. Roll your eyes back as if you were looking up into the top of your head.

10. Close your eyes.

11. You can repeat points 1–10, doing so 3, 6 or 9 times.

This completes the first phase of the power lock. As you practice, start combining each movement until you can smoothly complete all of the steps as a single locking movement.

LOCATING THE ENERGY POINTS ALONG THE SPINE

Locate and touch each of the key energy points on your spine. (On the next page see "**Energy Points or Centers Around the Spine.**") This will enhance your energy awareness as you move your energy into these points.

ENERGY POINTS OR CENTERS AROUND THE SPINE

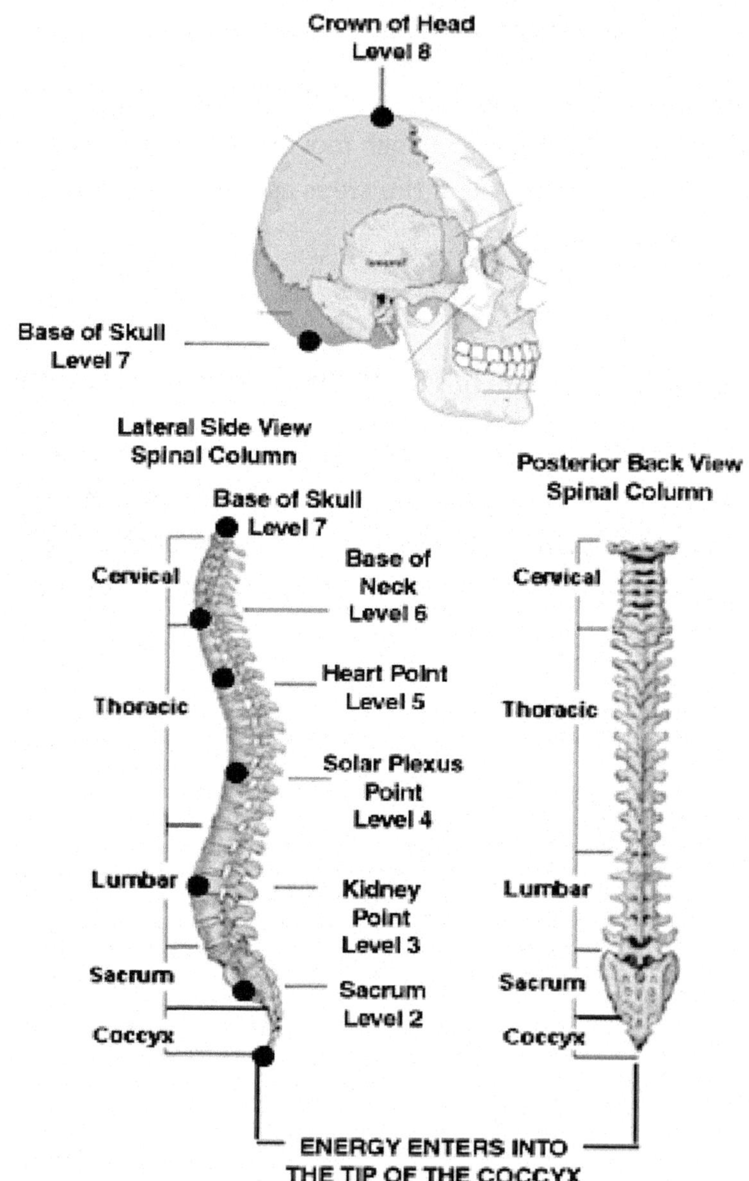

ORGASMIC BIG DRAW, LEVEL 1
THE PERINEUM CONNECTION

1. Repeat the Power Lock, part 1.

2. Exhale just a little.

3. Inhale, drawing a shallow breath.

4. Pull the aroused sexual energy into your perineum (the space in between your genitals and your anus).

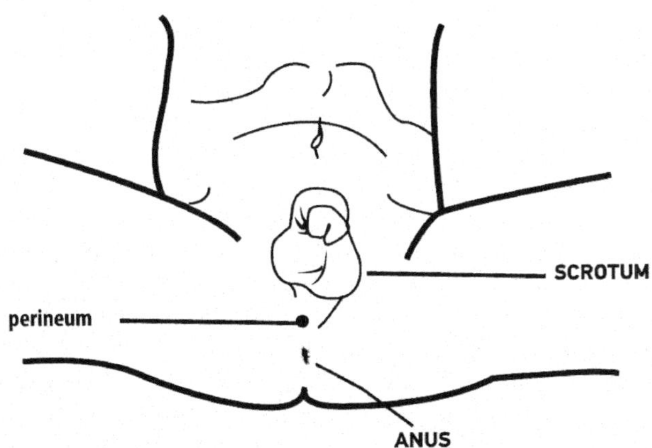

THE PERINEUM IS MIDWAY BETWEEN THE ANUS AND THE SCROTUM

5. Draw up your genitals and anus (slightly and lightly squeezing the anus). Use enough force to keep the area closed, but not so much as to cause discomfort (or run the risk of hemorrhoids).

6. Hold for a count of nine.

7. Exhale slowly through your nose.

8. Release and relax the muscles throughout your body.

9. Rest for 20 or 30 seconds.

10. Repeat this exercise (points 1–9) 3 times.

ORGASMIC BIG DRAW, LEVEL 2—THE COCCYX

After completing the Power Lock, part 1, continue to hold part 1 and add the Perineum Connection.

1. Repeat The Power Lock, part 1.
2. Exhale just a little.
3. Inhale, drawing a shallow breath.
4. Pull your aroused sexual energy into the perineum.
5. Exhale just a little.
6. Inhale, drawing a shallow breath.
7. Draw the sexual energy from the perineum to L1—the coccyx.
8. Hold for a count of nine.
9. Exhale slowly through your nose, releasing all the muscles throughout your body.
10. Rest for 20 or 30 seconds.
11. Repeat this exercise (points 1–10) 3 times.

ORGASMIC BIG DRAW, LEVEL 3—THE SACRUM

1. To begin—repeat the power lock, part 1—Now start with number 1, below:

2. Exhale just a little.

3. Inhale, drawing a shallow breath.

4. Pull the aroused sexual energy to your perineum. Take another short breath and complete the Orgasmic Big Draw. Repeat Level 1.

5. Exhale just a little.

6. Inhale, drawing a shallow breath.

7. Draw the sexual energy from your perineum into Level 1—the coccyx.

8. Exhale just a little.

9. Draw the aroused sexual energy from the coccyx up to the sacrum.

10. Hold for a count of nine.

11. Exhale slowly through your nose and release all the muscles throughout your body.

12. Rest for 20 or 30 seconds.

13. Repeat this exercise (1–11) 3 times.

ORGASMIC BIG DRAW, LEVEL 4—T11 (THE BACK OF THE SOLAR PLEXUS ALONG THE SPINE)

1. Repeat The Power Lock, part 1, and hold your in-breath.

2. Exhale just a little.

3. Inhale, drawing a shallow breath.

4. Pull the aroused sexual energy into your perineum. Take a shallow breath and complete the Orgasmic Big Draw. Repeat Levels 1, 2 and 3.

5. Exhale just a little.

6. Inhale, drawing a shallow breath.

7. Draw the sexual energy from your perineum into Level 1—the coccyx.

8. Exhale just a little.

9. Draw the aroused sexual energy from your coccyx to your sacrum.

10. Exhale just a little.

11. Inhale, drawing a shallow breath.

12. Draw the aroused sexual energy from your sacrum up to the T11 point (the back of the solar plexus along your spine).

13. Hold for a count of nine.

14. Exhale slowly through your nose, releasing all the muscles throughout your body.

15. Rest for 20 or 30 seconds.

16. Repeat this exercise (points 1–15) 3 times.

ORGASMIC BIG DRAW, LEVEL 5—
C7 (THE BASE OF THE NECK)

1. Repeat the Power Lock, part 1, and hold your in-breath.

2. Exhale just a little.

3. Inhale, drawing a shallow breath.

4. Draw your aroused sexual energy into your perineum. Take a shallow breath and complete the Orgasmic Big Draw. Repeat Levels 1, 2, 3 and 4.

5. Exhale just a little.

6. Inhale, drawing a shallow breath.

7. Draw the sexual energy from your perineum to Level 1—the coccyx.

8. Exhale just a little.

9. Draw the aroused sexual energy from your coccyx up to the sacrum.

10. Exhale just a little.

11. Inhale, drawing a shallow breath.

12. Draw the aroused sexual energy from your sacrum up to the T11 point (the back of the solar plexus along your spine).

13. Exhale just a little.

14. Inhale, drawing a shallow breath.

15. Draw your aroused sexual energy up from T11 (the solar plexus) to the C7 point (the base of the neck).

16. Hold for a count of nine.

17. Exhale slowly through your nose, releasing all the muscles throughout your body.

18. Rest for 20 or 30 seconds.

19. Repeat this exercise (points 1–18) 3 times.

ORGASMIC BIG DRAW, LEVEL 6—THE JADE PILLOW (THE BASE OF THE SKULL)

1. Repeat the Power Lock, part 1, and hold your in-breath.

2. Exhale just a little.

3. Inhale, drawing a shallow breath.

4. Draw your aroused sexual energy into the perineum. Take a shallow breath and complete the Orgasmic Big Draw. Repeat Levels 1, 2, 3, 4 and 5.

5. Exhale just a little.

6. Inhale, drawing a shallow breath.

7. Draw your sexual energy from your perineum to Level 1—the coccyx.

8. Exhale just a little.

9. Draw the aroused sexual energy from your coccyx up to your sacrum.

10. Exhale just a little.

11. Inhale, drawing a shallow breath.

12. Draw your aroused sexual energy from your sacrum up to the T11 point (the back of the solar plexus along your spine).

13. Exhale just a little.

14. Inhale, drawing a shallow breath.

15. Draw the aroused sexual energy up from the T11 point to the C7 point (the base of neck).

16. Exhale just a little.

17. Inhale, drawing a shallow breath.

18. Draw your aroused sexual energy up from the C7 point (base of the neck) to the "Jade Pillow" (base of the skull).

19. Hold for a count of 9.

20. Exhale slowly through your nose, releasing all the muscles throughout your body.

21. Rest for 20 or 30 seconds.

22. Repeat this exercise (points 1–21) 3 times.

ORGASMIC BIG DRAW, LEVEL 7—THE CROWN

1. Repeat the Power Lock, part 1, and hold your in-breath.

2. Exhale just a little.

3. Inhale, drawing a shallow breath.

4. Draw your aroused sexual energy into your perineum. Take a shallow breath and complete the Orgasmic Big Draw. Repeat Levels 1, 2, 4, 5 and 6.

5. Exhale just a little.

6. Inhale, drawing a shallow breath.

7. Draw your sexual energy from your Perineum to Level 1—the coccyx.

8. Exhale just a little.

9. Draw your aroused sexual energy from your coccyx up to your sacrum.

10. Exhale just a little.

11. Inhale, drawing a shallow breath.

12. Draw your aroused sexual energy from your sacrum up to the T11 point (the back of the solar plexus along your spine).

13. Exhale just a little.

14. Inhale, drawing a shallow breath.

15. Draw your aroused sexual energy up from the T11 point (the solar plexus) to the C7 point (the base of neck).

16. Exhale just a little.

17. Inhale, drawing a shallow breath.

18. Draw your aroused sexual energy up from the C7 point (the base of the neck) to the "Jade Pillow," the base of skull.

19. Exhale just a little.

20. Inhale, drawing a shallow breath.

21. Draw your aroused sexual energy up from the base of your skull (the "Jade Pillow") to your crown, the top of your head.

22. Hold for a count of nine.

23. Exhale slowly through your nose, releasing all the muscles throughout your body.

24. Rest for 20 or 30 seconds.

25. Repeat this exercise (points 1–24) 3 times.

Rest and feel your mind guiding your energy from your genital area up your spine and into your crown. You may also direct the energy around and down the front part of your body or spine. Allow this energy to circulate, and feel it encircling your body.

As you become more advanced, you'll find yourself using fewer muscle contractions (and less exertion) and more mind power. But remember, this will take time.

Practice, practice, practice—and doing so regularly and systematically—is the key. Do so and over time you'll have total command of your sexual skills.

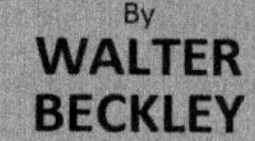

BECOMING AWARE

The techniques in this book are very powerful. For example, as you continue to master your sexual skills, you may start to feel a tingling—this sensation may be soft and warm or cool, like inner air-conditioning. It will flow in and through and around your body. You may also start to feel connected to the entire world or universe. And you may feel powerful waves of love flowing through you and a heightening of all your senses. You may start to see wonderful sights, hear beautiful music, taste sweet nectar and much more.

Because of its powerful possibilities, this book and the information it contains will **work best under the guidance of a qualified teacher**. Be sure to join the Sexual Power Training Network, an online service that assists men taking command of their sexual energies:

http://www.BuildingYourSexualStamina.com/member

FOR A MORE IN-DEPTH CONNECTION AND UNDERSTANDING, HEAR AND SEE OUR AUDIO AND VIDEO SERIES

When you join our Elite Membership site, you'll gain access to our audio and video library, which will enhance your learning experience. Plus, you'll get bonus information that will enable you to become a master in the art of lovemaking.

Go to:

http://www.BuildingYourSexualStamina.com/member

When you learn to master this section, you'll be ready to take command of all your sexual encounters.—Walter

17

TIPS FOR LONGER-LASTING SEXUAL EXPERIENCES

TIP 1—Always pee first.

You should always take time to urinate before sex. Don't worry about what your partner might think. You don't want to have a bad sexual experience because of too much pressure in your bladder. So stop and take the time to release yourself. Simply put, a full bladder pressing against a highly stimulated prostate equals premature ejaculations. Release the pressure and enjoy the ride.

TIP 2—Don't drink too much.

If you read the first tip, then you'll know why this is tip number 2. If you drink too much, the fluids will fill your bladder, which will press against the prostate and you'll find yourself facing a too-early ejaculation.

TIP 3—Relax.

Why should you relax when the whole point of sex is to get excited? Certainly, it's important for a man to feel his excitement. However, you need to pace yourself. Drawing out your excitement, making it last longer—that's the key. As you learn the art of relaxation, you'll come to grips with patience, which is a close cousin to relaxation and the father of power. When you learn to harness your power, there are no limits to how rough, soft, physically wild or rambunctious the two of you can be—if she wants or asks you to be.

TIP 4—Try this.

Once you are able take command of your sexual energy, experience the "relaxed power" method. After some long hard sexual intercourse (during which she'll have peaked several times—and you'll have had several major orgasms though not ejaculations), pause. Remain inside her, but pause, relax and be still. You may find yourself drifting off to sleep or going into a deep meditative state.

Many couples have reported seeing colors, feeling energy flow between them and even experiencing visions. While you are still hard and inside of the woman, together you can begin to relax and fall asleep. Your penis, while still inside her, will start to grow softer. When this happens, simply start moving or thrusting again inside of her. Also, when she feels your penis becoming softer, she may start to grip and pull you back in.

It's profoundly arousing, both sexually and emotionally, for a woman to drift off and awaken to realize that you are still connected and inside of her. Women simply love it.

TIP 5—Soft or relaxed entry.

If you find yourself so relaxed that you slip out of her, simply relax and gently reenter her. Then you can resume thrusting until you become fully erect again. This method of soft entry can be used in the beginning of sexual encounter as well as the end. However, you must be patient, and she must be very wet.

TIP 6—Caution!

Beware: Few women have had the experience of greatly extended sex; it could take some getting used to on her part. But most women love new experiences of this sort.

When you relax and drift off to sleep while still inside of your partner, check to be sure—if you're using a condom—that the condom doesn't slip off or that your partner hasn't accidentally pulled it off.

As a woman relaxes, her vagina will tighten, pushing your softened penis out. Don't worry if you feel this happening; start thrusting again until you become erect and once again you will be able to relax inside of her.

TIP 7—How hard should I be?

Become hard, enabling her to feel your power. Next, become firm, not too hard or too soft. You'll last longer, and she'll enjoy you even more. Your goal should be to gain the ability to shift from hard erections to firm erections—and to feel extreme comfort even when you become soft. Becoming soft is actually a ploy because with the techniques you have learned, you can easily become hard again. When you learn to play with the power of your erections, you'll start to feel extreme comfort and joy.

TIP 8—Tell her what you're doing.

When you decide to practice with a partner and if you're still working on the early stages of muscle contractions, be sure to tell her what you're doing. You don't want to surprise her, scare her or turn her off. Since some of these exercises call for what might (to those unfamiliar with them) appear to be fits or seizures, you should be sure to let her in on what you're up to.

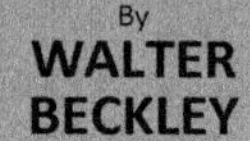

CONCLUSION

Now, having completed *9 Steps to Building Your Sexual Stamina*, you're well on your way to sexual mastery. You have completed the first level of sexual power training for men. This training should also help you be more aware of the possibilities that are available as a sexually conscious, skilled and sensitive lover. You've embarked on a new journey that I promise you will only get better as you hone your newfound skills.

As you continue referring back to and working the lessons in this manual, you'll keep expanding their value —and you'll continue fortifying your mind and body.

To further enhance your knowledge of lovemaking, I've set up a membership site where you can communicate with me and with other men and women who, like you, are learning sexual power training skills. You can learn more and join at:

http://www.BuildingYourSexualStamina.com/member

In this unique site you'll receive information on your next level of sexual training as well sexual health and fitness exercises and opportunities for interactive telephone seminars; special audios, videos and articles; and more.

I look forward to hearing about your progress and answering your questions. Don't feel that you have to figure this out on your own. I have trained around the world, and I bring this knowledge to you so you won't have to go without it or search to find it yourself.

QUESTIONS OR COMMENTS

Contact me at:
contact@BuildingYourSexualStamina.com

Wishing you the very best sexual experience ever!
—Walter Beckley

FOR A MORE IN-DEPTH CONNECTION AND UNDERSTANDING, HEAR AND SEE OUR AUDIO AND VIDEO SERIES

When you join our Elite Membership site, you'll gain access to our audio and video library, which will enhance your learning experience. Plus, you'll get bonus information that will enable you to become a master in the art of lovemaking.

Go to:

http://www.BuildingYourSexualStamina.com/member

You are invited to join my Elite Membership Program.

RESOURCE GUIDE

Suggested Readings:

The Healthy Living Game Plan: Book I
5 Sources of Silent Toxic Killers
That Attack Your Body and Your Loved Ones Everyday
http://www.OnlineDetoxProgram.com

The Healthy Living Game Plan: Book II
Super Charge Your Life: Turn Your Body's Stress Into Success—Look and Feel Better in 30 Days or Less—Learn How to Detoxify, Revitalize and Heal Your Body.
http://www.OnlineDetoxProgram.com

Web Sites and Services:

ELITE MEMBERSHIP PROGRAM
http://www.BuildingYourSexualStamina.com/member

PRIVATE COACHING PROGRAM
http://www.BreakthroughIntoGreatness.com

FOCUSED-POWER BREATHING METHOD®

http://www.BuildingYourSexualStamina.com/FPB

We offer instructional DVDs and CDs to enhance a deeper level of mastery over your breath.

RADIANT LIVING STORE

http://www.radiantliving.com/store.html

ONLINE DETOX PROGRAM

http://www.OnlineDetoxProgram.com

The cleaner your body is on the inside, the stronger your sexual energy will be—and the more fully that energy will be freed to grow and flow.

EASY EATING HEALTHY

http://www.EasyEatingHealthy.com

Discover how what you eat can increase and provide power, vitality, stimulation, stamina and enjoyment to your body, mind, emotions, relationships and sexual energy.

FOR A MORE IN-DEPTH CONNECTION AND UNDERSTANDING, HEAR AND SEE OUR AUDIO AND VIDEO SERIES

When you join our Elite Membership site, you'll gain access to our audio and video library, which will enhance your learning experience. Plus, you'll get bonus information that will enable you to become a master in the art of lovemaking.

Go to:

http://www.BuildingYourSexualStamina.com/member

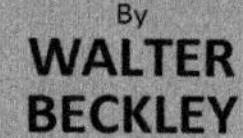

MAY YOU ENJOY ALL OF YOUR RELATIONSHIPS IN LIFE

Walter Beckley

THIS IS NOT THE END

JOIN NOW

FOR A NEW BEGINING

www.BuildingYourSexualStamina.com/member

CPSIA information can be obtained
at www.ICGtesting.com
Printed in the USA
LVOW01s1028190116
PP10484100001B/2/P